Magical Foods and The Mason Jar Life:
How to Make Plant-Based Meals in a Peaceful Kitchen

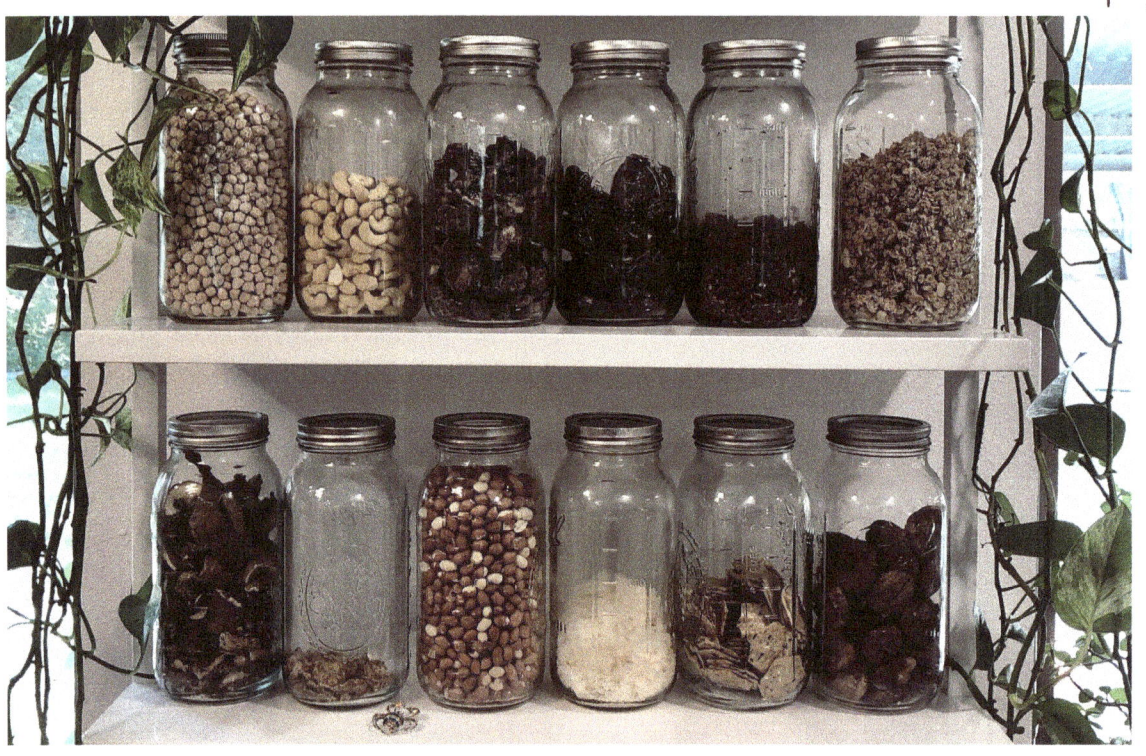

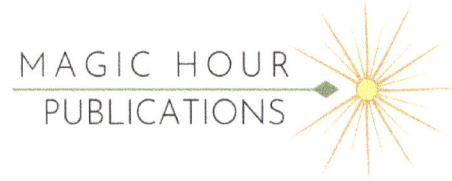

Copyright© 2023 Abe Louise Young

ISBN 978-0-9796082-5-4 (paperback)
ISBN 978-0-9796082-3-0 (ebook)
ISBN 978-0-9796082-2-3 (PDF)

Design by Caitlyn Perdue
Cover Design by Recspec Co

Table of Contents

WELCOME	06
EMBRACING MAGICAL FOODS	08
GRATITUDES & MEDITATIONS	11
ORGANIZING WITH JARS	13
Assemble Your Beautiful Jar Library	13
How to Order Your Jars	15
Labeling Jars	16
Use Jars for Snack Foods	17
Put Like With Like	17
COOK ONCE & EAT ALL WEEK	18
Step 1 Decide Menu and Soak Beans Overnight	19
Step 2 Make Plant-Based Milk	19
Step 3 Make Breakfast Jars	20
Step 4 Cook Lunch Beans	21
Step 5 Cook Lunch Pasta, Grains & Sauce	22
Step 6 Make Dinner Soup	23
Step 7 Prep Raw Vegetable Salads & Dressing	23
HOW TO BRING FOOD HOME	25
Shopping with Jars	25
Shopping for Larger Quantities	25
Shopping for Produce	26
Buy Vibrant Food	27
When to Buy Organics	28
Eat for Longevity	29
HOW TO ORGANIZE YOUR REFRIGERATOR	32
HOW TO ORGANIZE YOUR FREEZER	33
HOW TO KEEP A FOOD INVENTORY	34
HOW TO STAY HAPPY AND AVOID EATING JUNK	35
Defying Fast Food Urges Takes Effort	35
Eating Food Aligned with Our Values Creates Happiness	36
FOOD & WATER STORAGE FOR EMERGENCIES	38
RECIPES	40

Table of Contents Cont'd

PLANT-BASED MILKS — 41
- Soymilk — 41
- Oat Milk, Almond MIlk, Cashew Milk — 42
- Supplementing with Calcium — 42

BREAKFAST — 43
- Overnight Oats — 44
- Luxurious Chia Pudding — 45
- Pumpkin Tofu Pudding — 46
- Choose-Your-Own-Adventure Smoothie — 47
- Berry Green Smoothie — 50
- Peach Pie Smoothie — 51
- Chocolate Peanut Butter Smoothie — 52
- Magic Greens Smoothie — 53

PASTA, GRAIN & BEAN LUNCHES — 54
- Pasta with Red Lentil Tomato Sauce — 55
- Pesto Garbanzo Pasta — 56
- Peanut Saucy Noodles with White Beans and Scallions — 58
- Sumptuous Alfredo Pasta with Summer Peas — 59
- New Orleans Style Red Beans and Rice — 60
- Spicy Bean Macaroni Salad — 62
- Cranberry Quinoa with Green Peas — 63
- A Perfect Sandwich — 65

DINNER SOUPS & STEWS — 66
- Spicy Red Lentil Soup — 67
- Green Curry Tofu and Vegetables — 68
- African Peanut Yam Soup — 70
- Barley-Mushroom Soup with Tofu — 71
- Broccoli Cheeze Soup — 72
- Yellow Split Pea Soup (Matar Dal) — 73
- Black Bean, Kale & Butternut Squash Stew in the Slow Cooker — 74
- Classic Black Bean Soup — 75

RAW VEGETABLE SALADS & DRESSINGS — 76
- Coleslaw with Miso Ginger Tamari Dressing — 77
- Broccoli, Apples and Grapes with Apple Cider Vinaigrette — 78
- Shaved Brussels Sprouts with Cranberries and Almonds — 79
- Mason Jar Salad — 80

Table of Contents Cont'd

DELICIOUS ANYTIME	81
Crispy Baked Tofu	82
Falafel Patties	83
Cashew Queso	84
Bean Dip	85
Perfect Collards	86
Spicy Quick-Pickled Veggies	87
BREADS	88
Cornbread in a Cast Iron Skillet	89
Children's Bread	90
DESSERTS	91
Veronica's Haroset	92
Coconut Jicama Salad	93
Mango, Pomegranate, Blueberry Salad	94
Oatmeal Pecan Date Balls	95
Spiced Berry Sorbet	96
Cucumber Jalapeño Popsicles	97
Thumbprint Cookies	98
BODY CARE & CLEANING	99
Body Care Recipes	100
Cleaning Supply Recipes	102
ACKNOWLEDGMENTS	103
RECOMMENDED READING	104
ABOUT THE AUTHOR	105

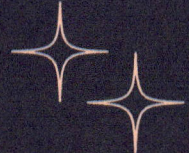

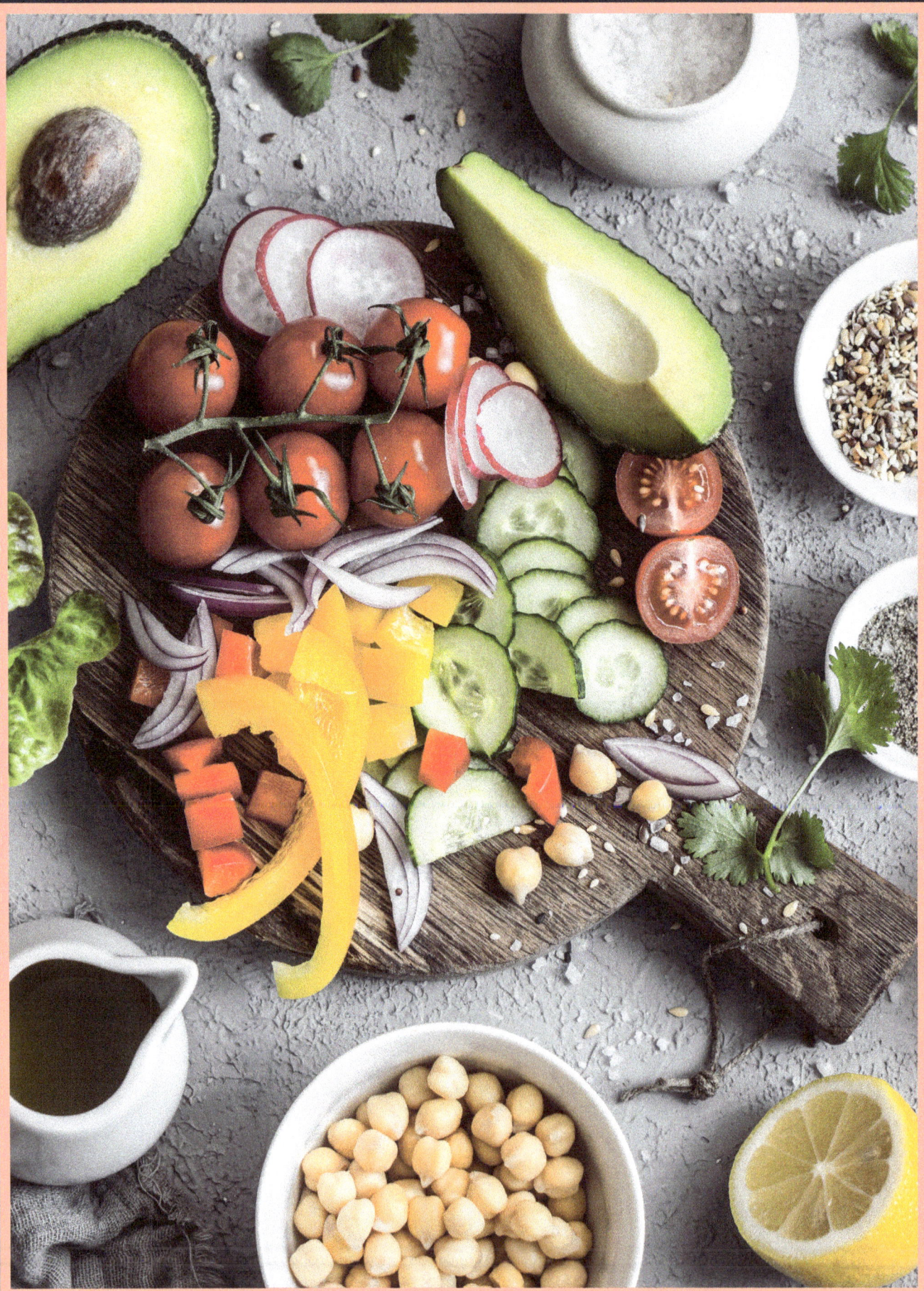

Welcome

Welcome! I'm thrilled to share my favorite recipes and the ways I've figured out to have a peaceful, fun, cheap and easy relationship with food. Cooking with the methods in this guide feels magical and artful—these foodways can deepen your sense of connection to yourself, other people, animals, and the Earth.

The strategies in these pages are proven methods for spending the least money for the most food, using the beauty of bulk goods stored in glass jars and cooking all your meals for the week, once a week.

I live in Austin, Texas where I grocery shop about once a month and get fresh produce from a farmers' market around every two weeks. I strive to only eat plant-based meals and I spend between $200 and $250 a month on food, buying mostly single organic ingredients.

I live alone and during the pandemic, preparing 3 meals a day for myself got hard. I found myself either in a fast-food drive-through line or spending $30 at a restaurant for dinner a little too often. I was also buying processed, packaged convenience foods and frozen meals, and it made me sad.

I've always stored my bulk goods in glass Mason jars, because I love to look at them. One day, I realized that the Mason jars had almost everything I needed for weeks of good meals. As long as I had fresh produce, I could go months without eating outside the house or ordering food delivery. It was time for a change.

I decided to figure out how to cook so that I had convenience, but with nourishing food I made at home. I wanted to feel like someone else was taking care of me—like someone had lovingly prepared me food and the fridge was full of easy, one-step meals. I never wanted to be hungry and lonely at the same time—I would be my own Mealtrain and Care Calendar.

I experimented with various ways of cooking, based on the ingredients in my jars. Now, I do one big batch cooking afternoon on Sundays for three to four hours. I prep meals for the whole week, and then spend a maximum of 10 minutes a day preparing food—just plating and heating it up. I feel taken care of, loved and nurtured by my own hands. I always feel good about what I'm eating.

Now, I set the table with a cloth placemat and napkin, light a candle, and put my phone away to eat. If I'm alone, I read a book or write in my journal. My meals are nutrient-dense rather than calorie-dense, packed with fruits, vegetables, legumes, whole grains, nuts and seeds, mushrooms, herbs and spices. I started by going 80%

plant-based, then slowly became about 95% plant-based. (I make exceptions for birthday cake, chocolate croissants and cultural or celebration food cooked by friends.) There's no such thing as perfection—any movement toward unprocessed food is movement in the right direction.

In this book, you'll learn:

- Easy Kitchen Habits and Methods
- A Plan to Cook Once and Eat All Week
- A Mason Jar System
- Pantry Shopping Lists
- Mindful Eating Magic
- Simple, Whole Food Plant-Based Recipes

Thanks for coming along! May your dining table be a happy place and may you have a lifetime of ease and joy in the kitchen.

Warmly,

Abe Louise

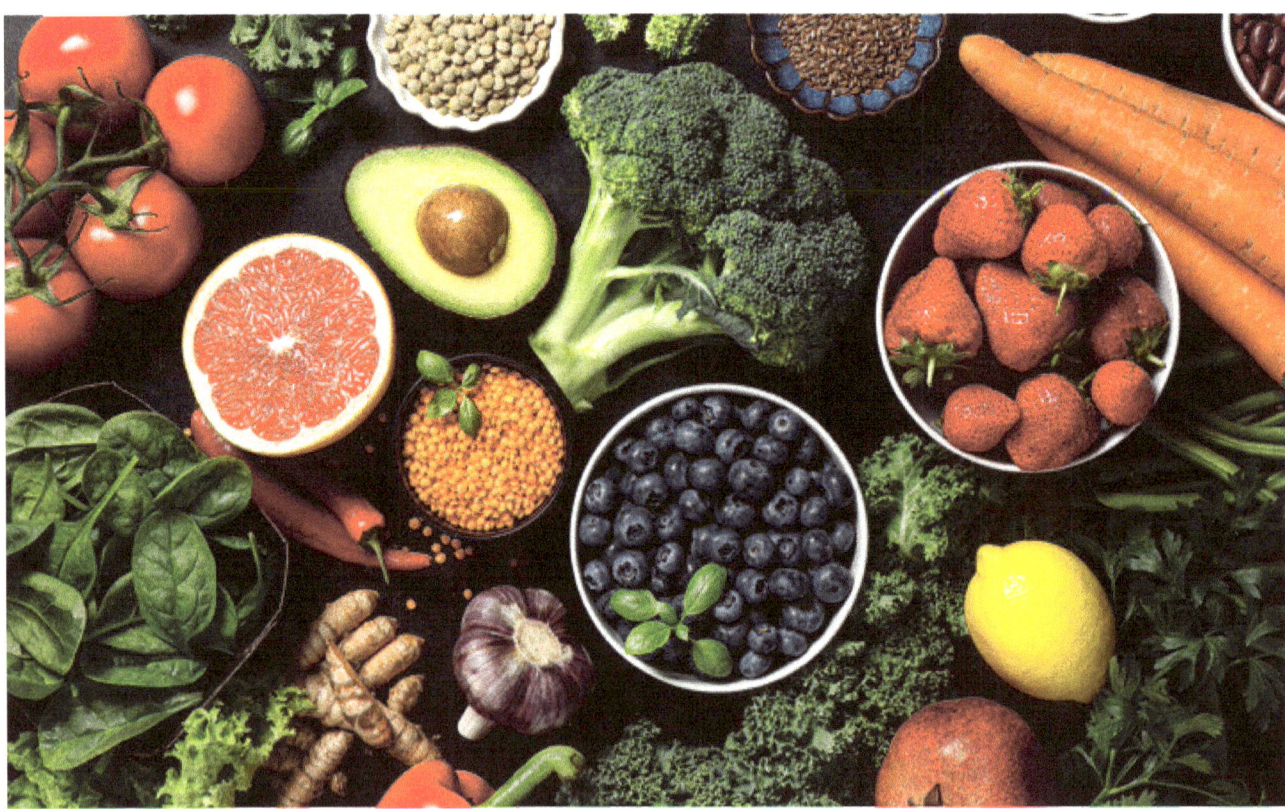

Embracing Magical Foods

Using plants in as close to the form as they grow out of the fertile Earth is magic. Holding a twisty sweet potato with whiskers and bulges and the whisper of its microbial soil is magic. Peeling it, skinning it, and seeing its bright orange body nearly vibrate with saturated color is magic.

Cooking with dry beans that are still so alive and full of potential that they will sprout a green leaf if soaked and bathed in water a few times is magic. Eating a seed, nut or grain that the Earth has evolved over tens of thousands of years to deliver concentrated energy is magic.

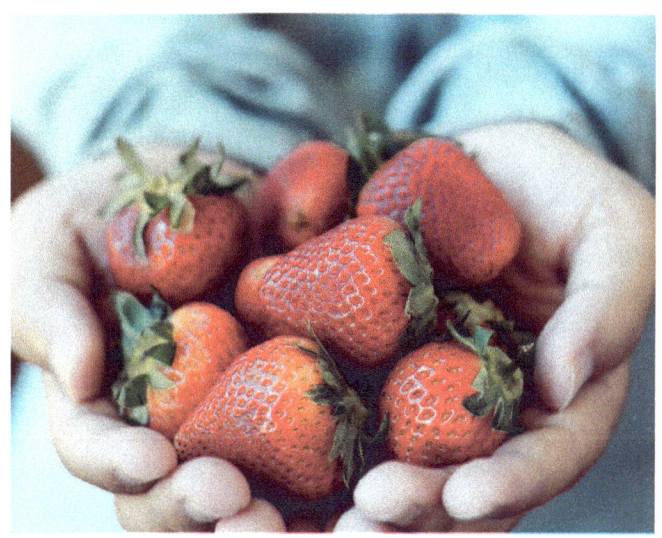

Spices and herbs are so full of active compounds and antioxidants that they're just delicious medicine, first medicine. Looking at the powdered brown, yellow, red and green spices in jars, I see a legion of quiet protectors.

Vegetables, fruits, whole grains, beans, nuts and legumes are most of we need to thrive, and that makes life simple. My basic plan for feeding myself with these magical foods is to eat nutrient-dense meals, raise my energy up to high gratitude, cook once, and eat all week.

I love knowing that these eating choices are also in alignment with my values and who I want to be in the world. I want to lower carbon emissions, protect the oceans, and slow climate change. Taking meaningful action on these issues with my daily life and kitchen is magic. Eating a plant-based diet means putting our beloved Earth's health first.

I aspire to be vegan, but I don't believe in perfection or purity. The middle way is usually more welcoming and sustainable. I don't cook or eat meat and I follow a vegetarian diet that's 90% dairy-free. A few times a month, I may eat something with small amounts of butter, cheese or eggs in it, usually baked goods. I want to protect the environment and protect animals from needless suffering with the majority of my choices. I don't see a reason to be draconian; my diet is intuitive, my primary commitments are upheld, and the net effect is positive! I invite you to also take small steps.

We can all make some positive shifts toward more plant-based eating, whether it's choosing plants one day a week or seven. Some people follow a flexitarian diet, some people practice VB5 (vegan before 5pm, so animal products are only consumed at dinner), or V5/2 (vegan on the weekdays and omnivorous on weekends). Other people learn plant-based recipes that taste like their animal-based favorites and slowly transition their kitchens over. Moving meat, fish and dairy from a main dish role to a condiment role, or off the plate completely, is a positive step for health and planet.

Whatever pattern works for you to integrate more plants onto your plate, you will reduce methane, carbon emissions, water pollution and animal cruelty. Your choice will protect the rainforest, ozone layer, oceans and rivers. It will give you better cardiovascular health and may mean a longer, more energetic lifespan. Any small step is a win! I celebrate you even reading this text and imagining your way to more plant-based meals! Imagination is a key ingredient for magic.

The kitchen system that I outline and detail in this guide helps me to maintain my commitments and experience food as easy, inexpensive, and fun. Here's are the rituals involved in how I do it. I don't expect anyone to suddenly prep all their meals and cook everything plant-based all at once. This set of steps is just what works for me. Draw from it or leave it, as you like, knowing you have the power to make food easy and fun in your world, too.

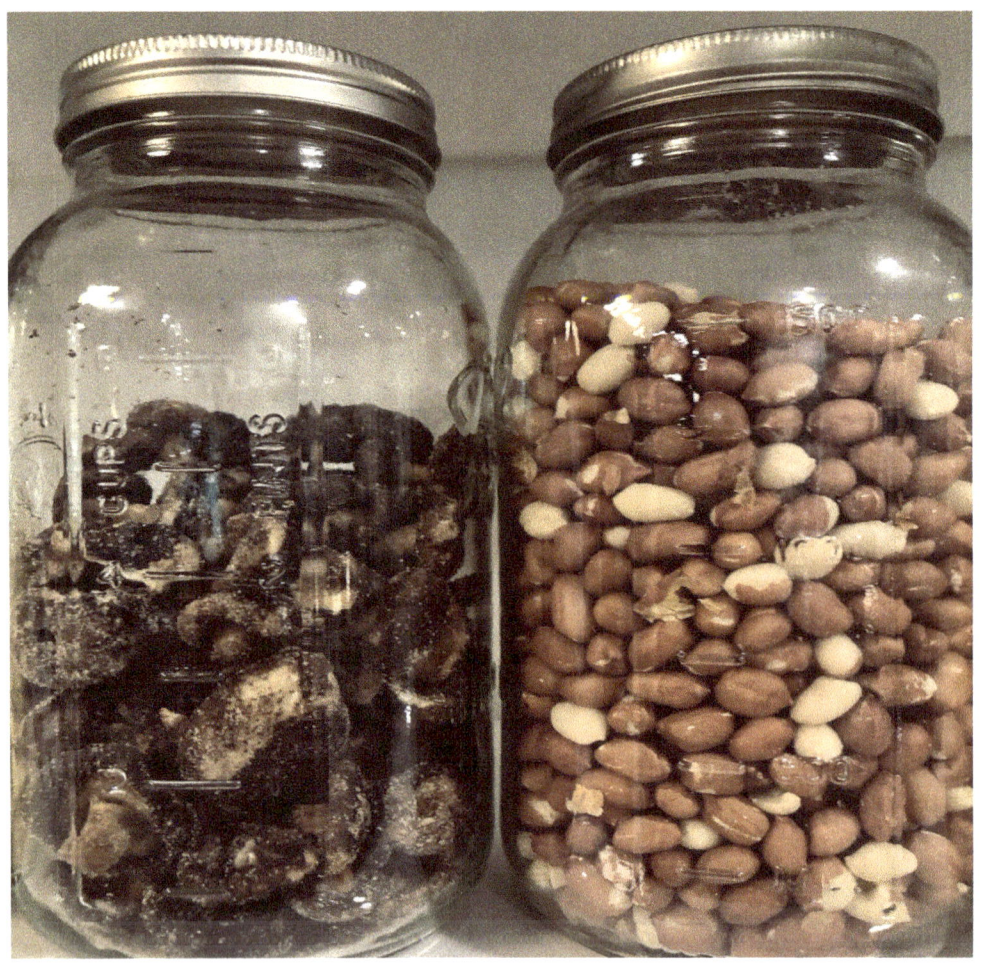

ON SATURDAYS

- I decide what to make for the next week. I look at my bulk jars to make sure I have the main ingredients and go to the farmer's market or grocery for produce if I need to.
- I wash all the empty food containers from last week.
- I pour the next weeks' beans in a bowl and cover them with water to soak before bed.

ON SUNDAYS

- I wake up, make coffee, and put on music.
- I think about my intentions for the week. I generate love and gratitude by thinking about all the hands involved in getting food to my kitchen. I feel my own great fortune to have plenty of nourishment and healthy food, and a home in which to cook. It could be otherwise.
- I cook for three or four hours using the seven steps you'll read about in this guide and overlapping the tasks. The kitchen is glorious disorder.
- I put all the food in glass containers and into the fridge and clean up.

By Sunday afternoon, my fridge is colorful as a quilt, full of containers of beautiful plant-based meals. I eat like a queen all week.

There's no doubt about the fact that grocery shopping, cooking a healthy diet for yourself or for a family, and cleaning up afterward is a lot of work. By putting all of that work into one or two days, you can free up the other days and nights to do more of what you love. You can also spread these different steps out over the week and have a rolling menu if you prefer.

NOTICE HOW IT FEELS

After doing the Mason jar life for a while, I feel happy, alive, creative and full of energy, like a sprout that will burst into green leaves when bathed in water and song.

I almost always have a full meal in my refrigerator, so I can set the table for any friends or loved ones who come to my home, light a candle, warm a colorful plate and a bowl of soup and feed them without any rush or stress.

As I cook over the weekend and see the beautiful meals filling up my fridge, I feel rich. When I'm out and get hungry in the world, I don't have cravings to stop at a fast-food joint or bakery. I think about all that luscious food waiting for me at home, and the hunger doesn't seem urgent. I used to panic at hunger pangs and treat it like an emergency. Now, it feels pleasurable, interestingly, like excited anticipation.

Gratitudes and Meditations

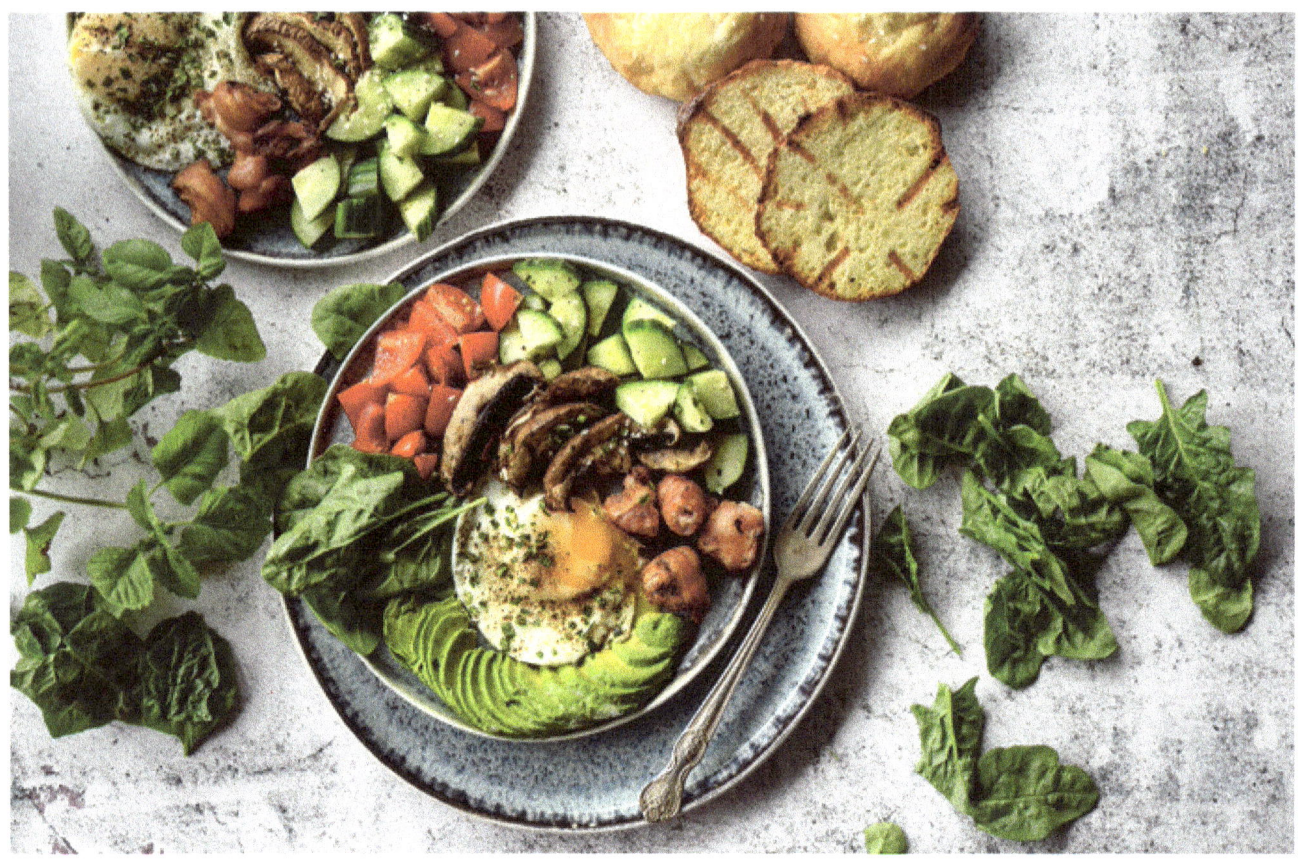

"If we look at our food for just half a second before putting it into our mouth and chewing it mindfully, we see that one string bean is the ambassador of the whole cosmos."

–Thich Nhat Hanh, from *The Mindfulness Bell #6*

MEDITATIONS

A meal feels sacred when we sit down to eat it and think about our gratitude and intentions. I like to light a candle at dinner and pause to read a poem or *The 5 Contemplations* by Thich Nhat Hanh.

Pausing to reflect, connect and experience gratitude before a meal is a nearly universal tradition on planet Earth.

Dogen, the 13th century Japanese monk who brought Zen Buddhism from China to Japan, included meal contemplations in monastic daily ritual. He called them The Five Reflections Recited Before Meals (Gokan no Ge). *The 5 Contemplations* below are a continuation of that tradition.

The 5 Contemplations

This food is the gift of the whole universe: the earth, the sky, the rain, the sun, numerous living beings and much hard, loving work. We thank all the people who have touched this food, including the farmers, the truckers, the shopkeepers, and the cooks.

We eat in mindfulness so as to nourish our gratitude.

May we keep our compassion alive by eating in such a way that reduces the suffering of living beings, stops contributing to climate change, and heals and preserves our precious planet.

May we only eat foods that nourish us and prevent illness.

We eat this food in order to be healthy and happy, to care for each other, and to live with understanding, love, and joy.

You can adapt these words and make them your own. A shorter, similar prayer offered by a friend reads,

We bless the soil, the sun, the minerals, the air, the water, and all the hands that touched this food. May we be nourished and well.

If you have eating companions, a short squeeze of hands around the table will deepen and ground the meal and make everyone feel included.

Mindful eating also means slowing down to notice the food, chewing slowly, not using distraction while eating, and following your body's signals about satiety. If you have companions, put away devices and talk. If you're alone, put away devices and simply appreciate the meal, or read or journal.

Many cultures nurture ritual practices based in the seasons using the four natural elements—water, fire, earth and air—in ceremony. These elements are often brought together alongside incantatory intention-setting to "spell" things into being. Every culture has its own variations on the sacred relationship between earth elements and words.

Cooking is the original magical ritual bringing water, fire, earth, and air together to sustain life. Any pot can be a cauldron if you light the fire, add the ingredients, think of your intentions, and stir. If you speak your gratitude and intentions aloud, it becomes active magic.

Organizing with Jars

The basis of a peaceful kitchen is food ingredients stored in Mason jars, a timeless system. I call this a jar library. The pleasure felt in looking at a raucous bookshelf spilling with novels and poetry waiting to be read can also be felt by gazing at a colorful shelf of food jars bursting with potential.

ASSEMBLE YOUR BEAUTIFUL JAR LIBRARY

Your jar library will reflect your unique tastes. Ingredients, especially spices, are highly subjective and culturally inflected—eat what you love! With a jar library filled with the food you adore you'll need to shop so much less often. You'll save time, mental space, and fuel.

Your jar library is a kitchen savings account. Filling a jar is an investment that will pay dividends in deliciousness, health and creativity. It's fine to start with a limited selection and add more jars over time as you build up ingredients. This keeps a kitchen organized. When I look at my jars, I feel incredibly fortunate and grateful.

These are the staples I keep in my jars for a fully stocked kitchen.

DRIED FRUIT
apples
apricots
cranberries
cherries
dates
figs
raisins

DRIED VEGGIES
dehydrated bell peppers
dehydrated garlic
dehydrated onions
dried mushrooms

NUTS
almonds
cashews
hazelnuts
peanuts
pecans
Brazil nuts
walnuts

SEEDS
chia seeds
ground flax seeds
hulled hemp hearts
pumpkin seeds
sesame seeds
sunflower seeds

GRAINS
barley
brown rice
brown rice pasta
farro
granola
popcorn
quinoa
rolled oats
whole wheat pasta

LEGUMES
black beans
chickpeas
lima beans
pinto beans

LEGUMES CONT'D
red kidney beans
red lentils
white (navy) beans
soybeans

NUT BUTTERS
peanut butter
almond butter
tahini (sesame seed butter)

SWEETS
candied ginger
chocolate almonds
chocolate espresso beans
cinnamon-sugar pecans
dark chocolate

PANTRY GOODS
almond flour
arrowroot powder
baking powder
baking soda
brown sugar
coconut milk
cornmeal
corn starch
nutritional yeast
oat flour
protein powder
turbinado sugar
white flour
whole wheat flour

BEVERAGES
chicory root powder
coffee
black tea
green tea
herbal tea

BOTTLED GOODS
agave nectar
canola oil
maple syrup
olive oil
sesame oil
soy sauce
vinegars (apple cider, balsamic, rice, white)

JARRED GOODS
(refrigerated)
curry paste
ketchup
miso
pesto
marmalade
jam
vegan mayonnaise
vegetable broth concentrate

CANNED GOODS
BPA-free canned beans
olives
diced tomatoes
tomato paste
tomato sauce

SPICES
allspice
basil
black cumin seed
black pepper
cardamom
cayenne pepper
cinnamon
chili powder
Chinese 5-spice
coriander
cumin
curry
dill
garam masala
garlic powder
ginger
mustard powder
nutmeg
onion powder
oregano
parsley
red pepper flakes
rosemary
sea salt
thyme
turmeric
za'atar

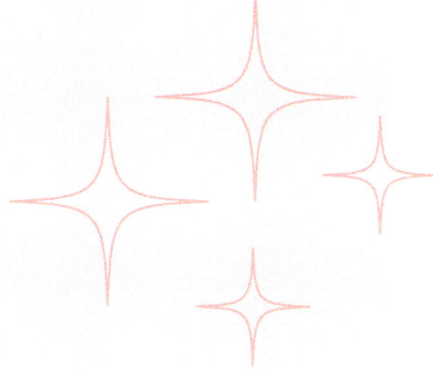

HOW TO ORDER YOUR JARS

Glass jars are the workhorse of the bulk ingredients system. They contain both the dry goods and raw ingredients, and many of the dishes and beverages you prepare each week in the fridge. I call my jars Mason jars, but Mason, Ball and Kerr jars are all good: they're just different brand names of equal value, with interchangeable lids. They work the same and are the same sizes.

To assemble and organize your jar library, the sizes you'll want are:

- Half gallon jars (64 oz)
- Quart jars (32 oz)
- Pint jars (16 oz)
- Half pint jars (8 oz)
- Spice jars (4 oz)

> Just make sure the jars you get are branded Ball, Kerr or Mason jars because knockoffs are not thick enough to stand the test of time.

You can buy jars online or at your local general store or supermarket. Buying them at a second-hand store is even better. Jars that you already have in your cabinets are best of all.

To contain all the foods listed in my jar library, as well as my cooked food, I use:

- 36 Half gallon wide mouth jars (64 oz)
- 36 Quart wide mouth jars (32 oz)
- 20 Pint wide mouth jars (16 oz)
- 10 Half-pint jars (8oz)
- 30 spice jars (4 oz)
- Snapware glass food containers in a variety of sizes

I'm a sucker for simplicity. I used to have both kinds of Mason jars: wide-mouth and regular mouth. But that meant having 2 different sizes of ring and top in a bag and digging around for the right size. I decided to replace all of my Mason jars with the wide-mouth variety, and I've been happy with that streamlining decision. My hand can reach right into the wide-mouth jars and their straight walls are easier to clean than regular-mouth jars, which are curved.

Gallon jars are nice to have for longer-term storage. I have six 1-gallon jars which keep backup supplies of beans and grains I use most and calm any apocalyptic anxieties. (Dried beans will last about 3 years in Mason jars that are opened and closed with use, but will last 25+ years in an airtight, dark container with an oxygen absorber added. Older beans just need a longer cooking time. I've eaten perfectly fine 5-year-old beans, adding an extra 20 minutes in the pressure cooker for tenderness.)

In the spice jar department, I splurged on hexagonal magnetic glass jars. They have the names of the spice stamped on the lid and make a gem-colored glass honeycomb on the fridge. Spices are ordered alphabetically.

The other set of glass items you'll need to contain your prepared food is a good selection of Pyrex or Snapware food containers, rectangular glass boxes with airtight lids with four tabs that snap down to keep them closed tightly. To keep them organized, store them with the lids on.

Using see-through glass containers for refrigerated, cooked food leads to less food waste because you'll keep the food that's ready to eat in visual sight in the fridge, and won't forget it.

I keep all of my working dry food jars on open shelves and have never had a problem with degradation due to light exposure. If you are storing ingredients for 2+ years, you'll want to keep them in a dark airtight container not exposed to light, but for the jars you use on a daily, weekly, or monthly basis, storing them in view is just fine.

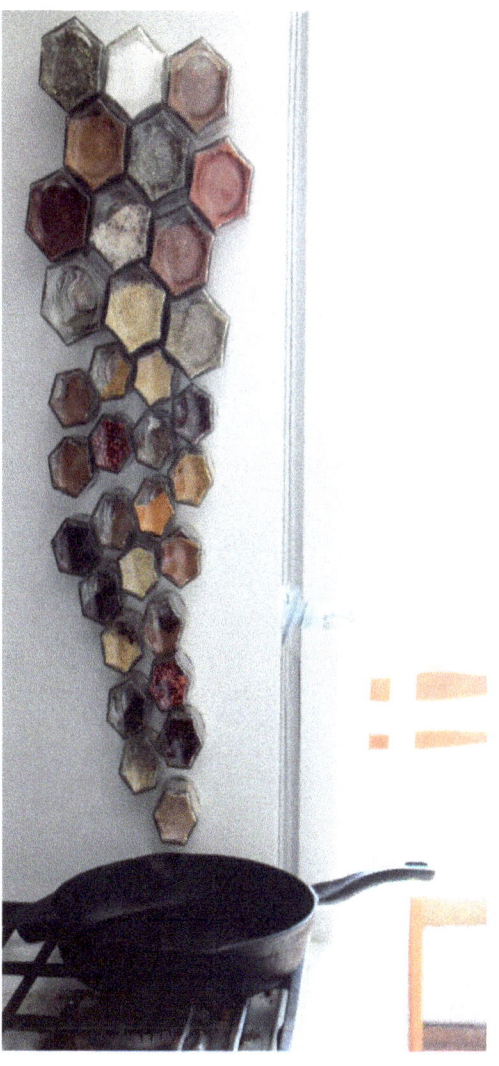

LABELING JARS

Over time you'll grow to know your ingredients at a glance but using labels can keep things organized. It can also inspire you to use ingredients if you're prompted by language. Seeing BARLEY on the jar may tickle your mind into looking for barley recipes.

To be honest, my affinity for glass jars began from my inability to tolerate seeing words on packaging. When I see brand names and marketing language, taglines and promo text, I read them over and over and repeat them in my mind–a kind of capitalist echolalia. I become frustrated that this empty language is taking up my awareness. I'd much rather look at pretty jars full of colorful, textured ingredients and their honest names and keep my mental quietude. For that reason, I only label tea jars and spice jars (you never want to confuse cinnamon and cayenne pepper!)

If you stash meals in the freezer, do label the container with the name of the dish and the date so you make sure to eat it within one to three months.

Ball Dissolvable Canning Labels, which dissolve in water, are pretty nifty. Labeling jars with more formal or permanent labels limits their usage, since you'll want to keep your jars in constant rotation for different ingredients, bulk and cooked.

> If you use dissolvable labels, dissolve and remove them under running water before putting jars in the dishwasher or they will gum up your filter.

USE JARS FOR SNACK FOODS

Use your jars for every kind of food that comes into the house. If I buy a treat for morale—like popcorn, cookies, or caramels—my rule for myself is to empty the bag into a Mason jar. This helps with portion control. If it stays in the bag, I'm likely to eat the whole bagful at one sitting because it just seems like it should be eaten. If I put it in a jar, I can more easily make choices about the portion, put a little in a small bowl and enjoy the snack for many days.

If something you're transferring to a Mason jar has cooking instructions that you want to remember, cut the instructions out of the box or bag it came in and stick them in the jar, right on top.

PUT LIKE WITH LIKE

When ordering jars in the kitchen, put like with like. Cluster all of your snack jars together in a snack altar. You can direct guests there to choose what they want to snack on, and always have something healthy at hand for yourself. Snack jars are stunning with food like dried peaches, apricots, figs, dates and berries, seasoned nuts and seeds, granola, crackers and sweet treats.

After separating snack jars from raw ingredients jars, order your dry raw ingredients into clusters: separate them into legumes, putting all your beans, peas and lentils together; grains, putting your quinoa, rice, cornmeal, couscous and other grains together; pastas, putting your spaghetti, soba noodles, brown rice spirals and other shapes together; baking goods, putting your flours, sugar, baking soda and powder together; and teas, coffee, and spices.

If they're on display, visitors will likely remark over them and praise their beauty, because raw ingredients in jars inspire people the same way fresh art supplies do.

Cook Once and Eat All Week:
A Peaceful Kitchen System

Cooking multiple meals at one time is the heart of a simplified kitchen. It takes the drudgery out of food prep and fills your fridge with delicious options for every meal. You never have to get hungry or worry about what's for breakfast, lunch, or dinner when you don't have the energy or wherewithal to cook. It's already done.

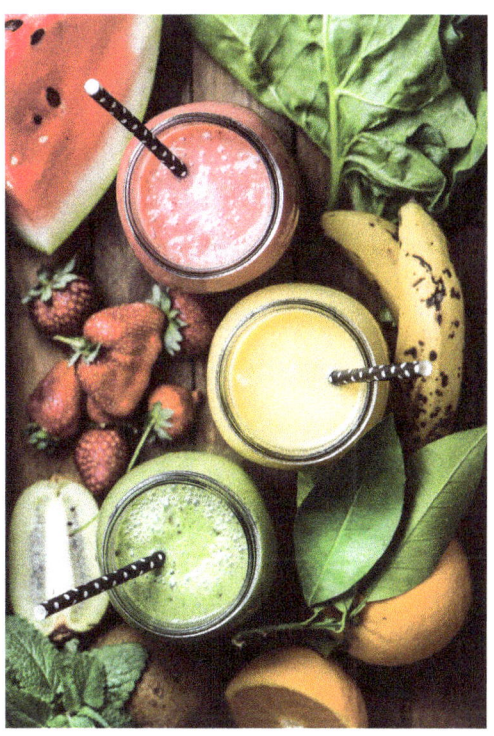

I'm someone who gets decision fatigue easily. Reducing the number of daily decisions helps me focus on making choices in my creative endeavors. Not breaking my flow state to figure out what to cook or eat while I'm working supports productivity and happiness.

As described earlier, I decide on Saturday what I want to eat for the next week and shop if necessary. I cook on Sundays and don't have to make any more food decisions for the rest of the week. With efficient batch cooking, those decisions are already made and I'm happy about them. This concentrated cooking time lets me use my daily energy making decisions about words, sentences, colors, textures, and how to take care of people—while still eating the most healthful diet around.

It's fun to do meal prep and batch cooking with a loved one or friend. Listening to music makes the food taste better. You can do this cooking in one morning or afternoon or spread it over the weekend or week on a rolling basis at your leisure. I find it easiest and most efficient to just do it all at once. If you don't have the time or energy to follow seven steps, choose just a few steps that will make your week more relaxed, like breakfast jars, or a dinner soup, and give that a try.

1. Decide Menu and Soak Beans Overnight
2. Make Plant-Based Milk
3. Prep Breakfast Jars
4. Cook Lunch Beans
5. Cook Lunch Pasta, Grains & Sauce
6. Cook Dinner Soup
7. Make Raw Veggie Salads & Dressing

Let's look at the system in a little more detail.

STEP 1. DECIDE MENU AND SOAK BEANS OVERNIGHT

On Saturday, decide your menu by looking through cookbooks and your pantry. Go to the store or farmer's market for any elements you don't already have in your jar library, pantry, fridge and freezer.

On Saturday night, soak any beans you'll need for your plant milk, lunch dish or dinner soup. Pour the beans into separate bowls and fill the bowls with water, covering the beans with an extra 2 or 3 inches of water. If your house is warm, soak beans in the fridge.

If you forget to soak overnight, you can do a quick soak: boil beans in water for 3 minutes, then cover pot and soak for 4 hours. Always rinse beans after soaking and discard the extra water, rather than cooking with it.

If you're going to make nut milk or a cashew-based sauce, also soak the nuts on Saturday night. Soaking beans and nuts is a slow and ordinary meditation practice; it's beautiful to see them swell and wake up.

STEP 2. MAKE PLANT-BASED MILK

On Sunday morning, I first make soymilk, a half-gallon jar full at a time. No matter how rushed or ungrounded I may be in the week, I know this sweet, frothy, honest earth milk will give me a dose of comfort and protein.

> One cup of unsweetened soymilk has 105 calories and 7 grams of protein.

This is the first action on Sunday because you'll probably need plant milk to use in later recipes, the breakfast jars and dinner soup. Homemade plant-based milk is easy, cheap, and healthier than what you get in the store—it does not have preservatives, salt, sugar or added thickeners such as carrageenan or xanthan gum. (It's also fine to use store-bought plant milk to save time and simplify things.)

I use a plant-based milk maker called the Soyabella that produces a quart of milk in 30 minutes. It can also make oat milk, rice milk, almond milk, cashew milk, hemp milk and every other kind of plant milk.

Recipe:

Plant-Based Milk, p. 41

STEP 3. MAKE BREAKFAST JARS

Make your choice of the following: Overnight Oats, Chia Pudding and Pumpkin Tofu Pudding, or a Smoothie. For each, you'll combine ingredients with plant-based milk.

I like to make 2 jars of overnight oats, 2 jars of chia pudding or pumpkin tofu pudding, and 2 smoothie jars at once. Except for the smoothie, these go in pint glass jars. Each morning, I eat one of the oats or chia pudding jars and drink half a smoothie. Do whatever combo appeals to you!

You can prep smoothies directly into the jar of a bullet blender (the easiest method) or into a quart Mason jar that you'll pour into a high-speed blender, or into Ziploc bags that you freeze. The bullet blender is by far the easiest.

When you prep smoothie jars, each recipe/jarful has 2 portions of smoothie. I drink half one day, and half the next day, with a stainless steel straw. If you use a bullet blender, consider investing in a few extra blender jars and jar tops so you can prep, blend and drink each smoothie in one jar and prep multiples ahead of time with no extra dishes to wash.

Related Recipes:

Overnight Oats, p. 44
Luxurious Chia Pudding, p. 45
Pumpkin Tofu Pudding, p. 46
Choose Your Own Adventure Smoothie, p. 47
Berry Green Smoothie, p. 50
Peach Pie Smoothie, p. 51
Chocolate Peanut Butter Smoothie, p. 52
Magic Greens Smoothie, p. 53

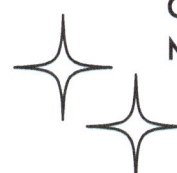

STEP 4. COOK LUNCH BEANS

Cook two cups of dry beans to have tender beans all week long. This makes 6 cups cooked, which is ideal for one person for a week. A pressure cooker makes quick work of it. You can also cook your beans on the stove in a pot; I've included both sets of directions in recipes.

I like to throw a few things in with beans:

- 1 Tablespoon garlic (fresh, minced or dehydrated)
- a bay leaf
- a piece of seaweed (nori or wakame)
- a splash of olive oil
- a low-sodium bouillon cube

Soak your beans overnight if you can. If you forget, use a pressure cooker/Instant Pot and just add six to ten minutes of extra cook-time.

When your beans are done cooking, taste them to make sure they're tender all the way through—if not, cook a little longer. Cooking time depends on the age of the beans. Salt your beans at the end, not at the beginning, otherwise their skins will get tough.

I love to cook dry beans because it's inexpensive, delicious, and waste-free, but there are plenty of times I used canned beans—especially when I'm tired, traveling or short on time. There's absolutely nothing wrong with cooking with canned beans. If saving time is your priority over saving money, use canned beans.

Look for low sodium or salt-free beans and be sure to drain and rinse any beans that come in a can. Regular canned beans have about 350 mg of sodium, which is not heart healthy. Rinsing the beans cuts that to about 165 mg of sodium—much better.

If cost is your primary consideration, dry beans cost about 1/4 the price of canned beans.

Here are some helpful rules of thumb for using dry beans.

- 1 cup of dry beans = 3 cups of cooked beans
- 1/3 cup of dry beans = 1 cup of cooked beans
- 1 pound of dry beans = 2 cups of dried beans or 6 cups of cooked beans

Here are some tips for comparing dry beans to canned beans.

- 1/2 cup of dry beans = one 15-oz. can of cooked beans
- 1.5 cups of cooked beans = one 15-oz. can of beans

All of the bean recipes in this book are written to refer to both cooked beans and canned beans. Cooking beans in larger quantities and keeping a variety in the freezer will give you an excellent stock to draw from.

Bean recipes are very flexible and forgiving. You can usually interchange similar-sized beans in a recipe to your heart's content. For example, you can use pinto beans instead of kidney beans, or garbanzo beans in place of navy beans in a recipe. You may need to adjust the cook time slightly. Experiment and have fun!

STEP 5. COOK LUNCH PASTA, GRAINS & SAUCE

Lunch in this system often consists of whole grain pasta, beans, and a delicious sauce–plus seeds and greens thrown on top and any veggies you want to add.

While your beans are cooking, boil water and cook 1 bag of whole grain pasta on the stove. Tinkyada Brown Rice Pasta, Banza Chickpea Pasta and 100% whole wheat pasta are all good. These just boil, but every noodle is different–follow the recipe on the bag.

In a big bowl, mix your pasta or grains, beans, and a sauce. You can make your own sauce or use a jarred sauce like pesto sauce or peanut sauce to save time.

Then garnish it with nuts and seeds and anything else that strikes your fancy. Pour this into a big glass snap-lock container. You have lunch or dinner for the week! When you take out a portion and heat it up, add some leafy salad greens after heating to increase the green quotient.

If you have more lunch than you will eat in a week, put a portion or two into the freezer, labeled with the date and name of the dish.

Related Recipes:

    Pasta with Red Lentil Tomato Sauce, p. 55
    Pesto Garbanzo Pasta, p. 56
    Peanut Saucy Noodles with White Beans and Scallions, p. 58
    Sumptuous Alfredo Pasta with Summer Peas, p. 59
    New Orleans Style Red Beans and Rice, p. 60
    Spicy Bean Macaroni Salad, p. 62
    Cranberry Quinoa with Green Peas, p. 63
    A Perfect Sandwich, p. 65

STEP 6. MAKE DINNER SOUP

Having soup for dinner lets your body slow down and not work so hard as you get close to sleep and inactivity time.

Slow cook, stove cook or pressure cook your dinner soup. Make a half-gallon jar of soup to eat for dinner all week.

If you are hungry when evening comes and the soup and raw veggie salad don't fill you up enough, bake some tofu, cook up a mess of collard greens, or make crackling cornbread or children's bread to accompany your meal.

Related Recipes:

- Spicy Red Lentil Soup, p. 67
- Green Curry with Tofu and Vegetables, p. 68
- African Peanut Yam Soup, p. 70
- Barley-Mushroom Soup with Tofu, p. 71
- Broccoli Cheeze Soup, p. 72
- Yellow Split Pea Soup (Matar Dal), p. 73
- Black Bean, Kale & Butternut Squash Stew, Slow-Cooked, p. 74
- Classic Black Bean Soup, p. 75
- Crispy Baked Tofu, p. 82
- Falafel Patties, p. 83
- Perfect Collards, p. 86
- Cornbread in a Cast Iron Skillet, p. 89
- Children's Bread, p. 90

STEP 7. PREP RAW VEGETABLE SALADS & DRESSING

Chop up some hard raw vegetables, such as half a cabbage, half a head of cauliflower and a few carrots for your raw vegetable slaw. Prep a dressing in the blender and mix the slaw with the dressing. Fill one glass snap-lock box with your dressed slaw.

> If saving time is your priority, you can buy a bag of already-chopped slaw at the grocery.

In another glass container, prep your salad greens.
I prefer to buy baby leaves like baby arugula, baby kale, and baby spinach because they save time chopping and tearing up pieces. They are also tender and adorable.

You can mix these greens with your slaw at the time of eating if you like. Keep them separate in the fridge. Since the slaw is made of hard vegetables, it will keep just fine with dressing for a week in the fridge, but that would make a green salad wilt and be unappetizing. Dress a green salad right before eating it and add any softer fruits like cucumber and tomato at that time.

When you get home with fresh leafy greens, transfer them to an airtight glass snap-lock box right away, putting a paper towel on top and on bottom of the box to absorb moisture. The greens can stay fresh for 7 days.

Related Recipes:

    Coleslaw with Miso Ginger Tamari Dressing, p. 77
    Broccoli, Apples and Grapes with Apple Cider Vinaigrette, p. 78
    Shaved Brussels Sprouts with Cranberries and Almonds, p. 79
    Mason Jar Salad, p. 80
    Spicy Quick-Pickled Veggies, p. 87

That's it! Your entire week is taken care of. If you have a hankering for dessert, have fresh fruit or dried fruit and dark chocolate from your snack jars. If inspired, make a dessert (see p. 91).

Once you put everything into its glass containers and inside your fridge, marvel at the beauty and thank yourself.

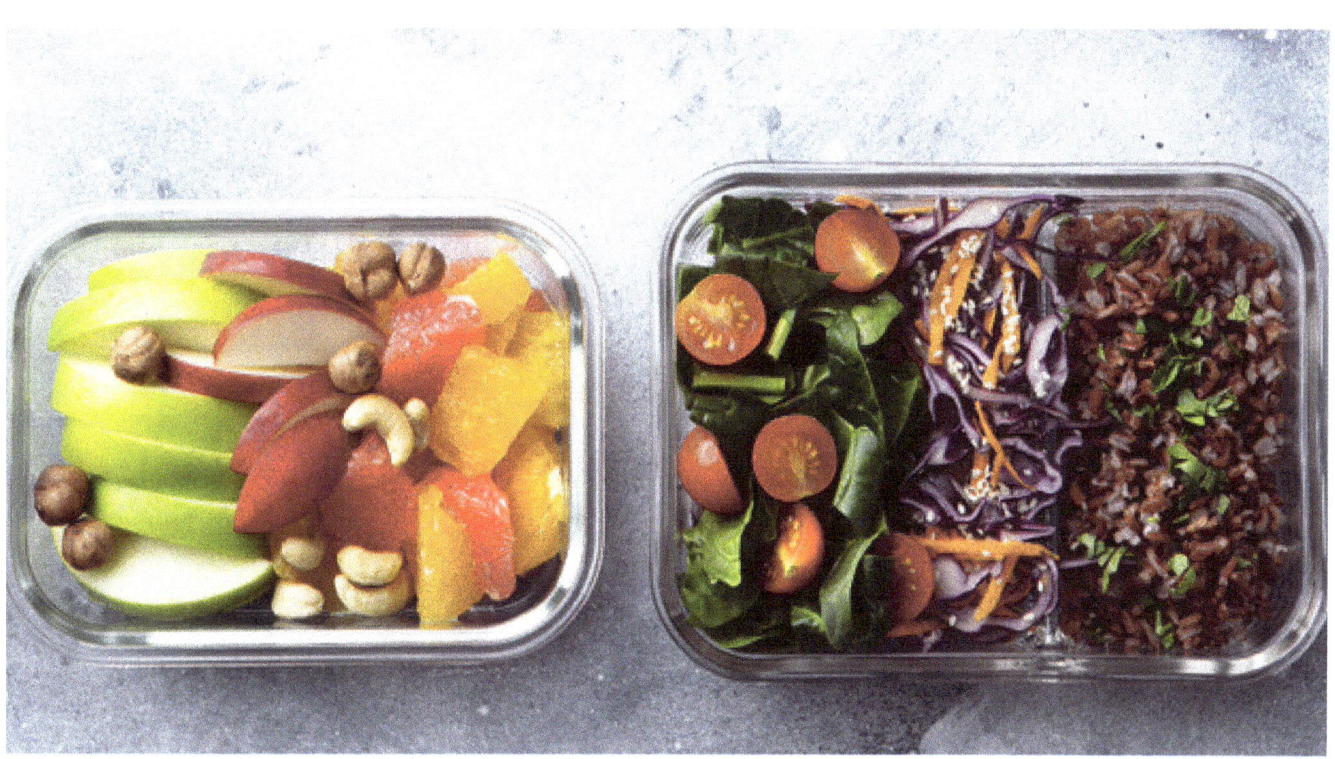

How to Bring Food Home

With Mason jars as your kitchen storage system, once you have a well-stocked jar library, you'll be going to the store far less often. You can store so much more food than you could ever keep in cans, bags and boxes—and you'll be less tempted to make impulse purchases.

When you do go to the store, you'll stay on the outer edges with produce and bulk goods, rather than the interior aisles where food gets ultra-processed. Ideally, there is a natural foods co-op in your town or a local grocery, or a place to buy bulk organic goods free from packaging, and local, organic fruits and veggies.

If you don't live nearby a store with a good organic bulk section, you can also use the internet or a discount membership store like Costco to buy dry goods in larger quantities. I've added the best and cheapest sources for bulk ingredients online below.

To fill your jars, buy bulk goods in the largest quantities you can comfortably afford and store in the space available to you.

> Spices can lose potency over time. Stick to half-pint jars or smaller for spices.

SHOPPING WITH JARS

I bring gallon, half-gallon, quart and pint glass jars to the natural foods co-op. I weigh the empty jars and write the tare (empty) weight on the bottom. The checker subtracts that jar weight from the total weight when the jar is full of ingredients.

This is the best way to get the best price per pound for bulk goods. It also avoids plastic and packaging completely. If you don't want to bring jars to the store, you can also package the dry goods in the free paper or plastic bags provided by the store and transfer to jars later. Be sure to write the 2- or 3-digit item bulk code on the bags for the checker.

Any natural foods co-op has bulk goods, and you don't need to be a member of a co-op to shop there. Organic red lentils in bulk at my co-op are $2.79/lb. They are also packaged on the aisle from various brands, starting at $3.79/lb. On Amazon, a pound of organic red lentils today ranges from $3.99 to $7.95/lb. This is the same pound of food, in different clothes. The bulk aisle will almost always be cheapest.

SHOPPING FOR LARGER QUANTITIES

Another way buy inexpensive ingredients is to buy in larger quantities. The larger the quantity, the small the price per unit, usually. You can do this easily at a discount membership store like Costco or Sam's Club. Just stay focused and ignore *all* the palate-tempting processed snack foods!

For organic dry goods, you can get excellent value at a bulk online retailer like bulkfoods.com, which is responsive to customers and has the lowest prices I've found. You might also find good deals and new ingredients to try at Asian and Middle Eastern grocery stores.

Wherever you source your bulk goods, transfer them to airtight storage when you get them home. Fill up all your glass jars. If you get larger bags of goods, such as 3-lb, 5-lb or 10-lb bags of beans or grains, close them up tightly and stash them in an airtight plastic tub kept dark and cool in the back of a closet.

SHOPPING FOR PRODUCE

Farmer's markets are the most soul-nourishing place to buy fresh fruits and vegetables! Joy cascades in those spaces and community bonds are deeply watered. If you aren't on a tight budget, the cost is well worth it for the experience and human connections.

Local farms also offer CSA boxes, which stands for Community Supported Agriculture. This is the original subscription box concept! You pay in advance for a season (buy a "share") and get a weekly or biweekly cardboard box filled with just-picked fruits and vegetables grown by a farm or farm collective near you. It's simple and humble, but the impact is profound and the produce is divine.

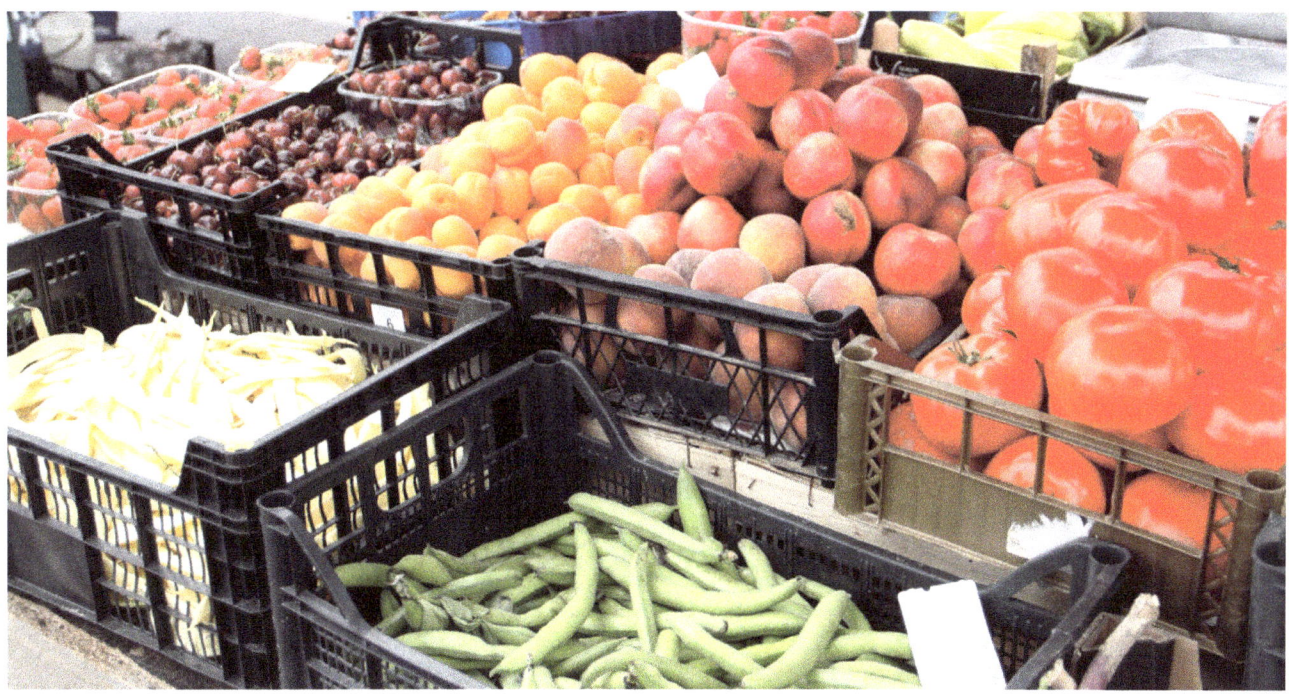

If buying directly from a farmer isn't in the cards for you, it's also just fine to get your fruits and veggies at a nearby grocery store. I bring a big woven basket to put produce in, rather than a reusable bag, so tender things don't get stacked on top of each other.

BUY VIBRANT FOOD

When shopping for produce, eat the intensely-colored rainbow. There's an easy way to make selections between different varieties of fruits and veggies: look for the darkest pigmented hue. In addition to your daily leafy greens, look for the most vibrantly, darkly colored versions of fruits and vegetables—the bright reds, blues, and purples. They will have the most anti-inflammatory antioxidants and anthocyanins, which are their disease-preventing compounds.

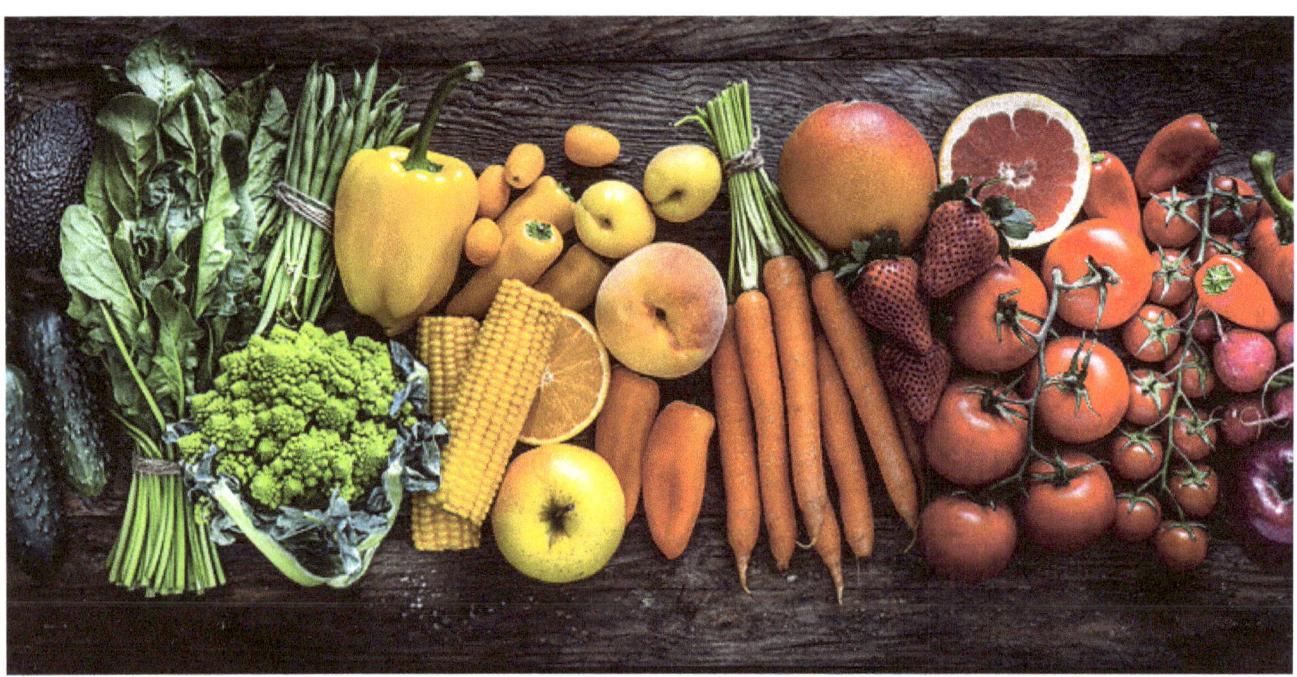

For disease prevention and fighting illness, red or purple cabbage is better than green cabbage; red onions are better than yellow or white onions; red or black grapes are better than green grapes; cranberries are better than raisins; blueberries are better than bananas; red quinoa is better than white quinoa, and so on. All fruits and veggies are good fruits and veggies but reach for the most vibrant first.

Likewise, cruciferous greens (arugula, cabbage, collard greens, kale, turnip greens) have more disease fighting power than non-cruciferous greens (lettuce, Romaine lettuce, spinach, etc.). This is because of a potent phytochemical called sulforaphane that gives cancer cells a death blow. Broccoli, cauliflower, and brussels sprouts also deliver this miracle compound. The most cancer-preventative food science has yet discovered is garlic and close second is broccoli sprouts, the food highest in sulforaphane. I keep a jar of broccoli seeds growing into sprouts on the windowsill and blend them daily in green smoothies because I love this planet and I want to stick around.

WHEN TO BUY ORGANICS

Buying organic ingredients is important for health, but it does raise the cost of groceries. How do we know which are most important to buy? An organic certification doesn't necessarily mean the food is good for you—it could be ultra-processed organic food laden with salt, added sugar and added fat. Ignore whatever words and images are on the front of a package and turn it over to look at the nutritional info on the back. That will give direction. In terms of produce, however, there's a great list to follow.

If it's not in your budget to buy all of your produce organic, try to avoid the Dirty Dozen: the twelve most pesticide-saturated foods. This list is released each year based on annual testing by the Environmental Working Group. If you can afford to, buy organics instead of these chemical-laden conventionals, ranked in order of pesticide load:

1. strawberries
2. spinach
3. kale, collard and mustard greens
4. peaches
5. pears
6. nectarines
7. apples
8. grapes
9. bell and hot peppers
10. cherries
11. blueberries
12. green beans

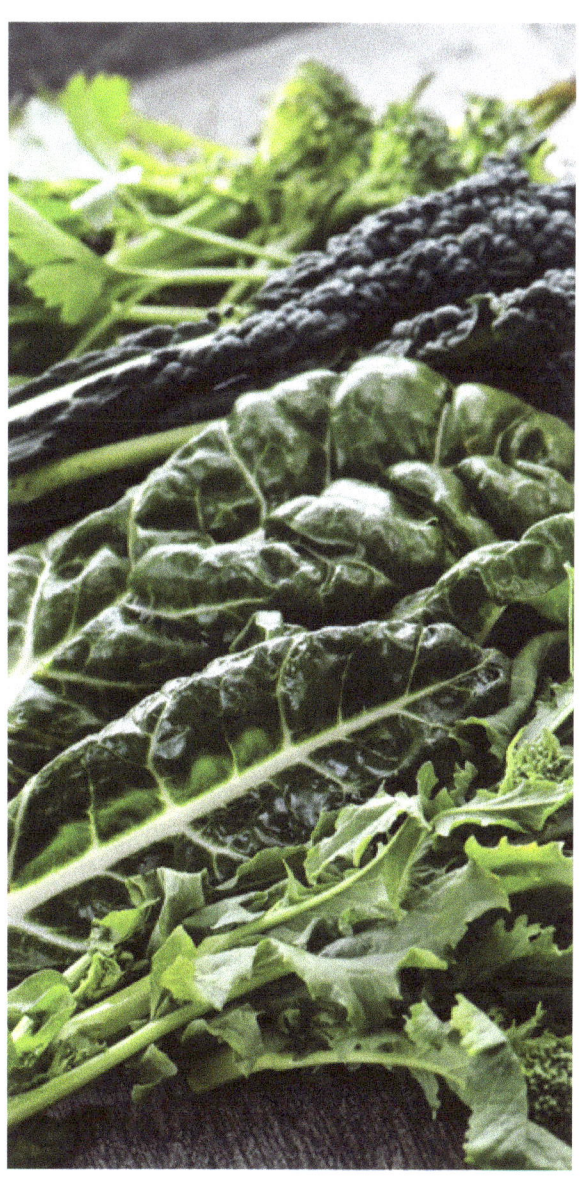

Conventional produce can come with residues of more than 45 different chemical pesticides. When you buy conventional produce, a very effective way to remove the cocktail of contaminants is a simple ingredient already in your pantry: baking soda.

All fresh produce needs to be washed, and a 2017 study on apples found that a baking soda and water soak removed all pesticide residue. Just put your produce in a bowl, cover it with water and add one teaspoon of baking soda for every two cups of water. Agitate it then allow it to sit for fifteen minutes. Drain the murky water off, rinse the produce, and put it in an airtight container. Safe and clean!

Conventional produce items that carry the *least* pesticide loads, and thus are safer to buy non-organic versions of, include:

1. avocados
2. sweet corn
3. pineapples
4. onions
5. papaya
6. sweet peas (frozen)
7. asparagus
8. honeydew melon
9. kiwi
10. cabbage
11. mushrooms
12. mangos
13. sweet potatoes
14. watermelon
15. carrots

These are known as the "clean fifteen."

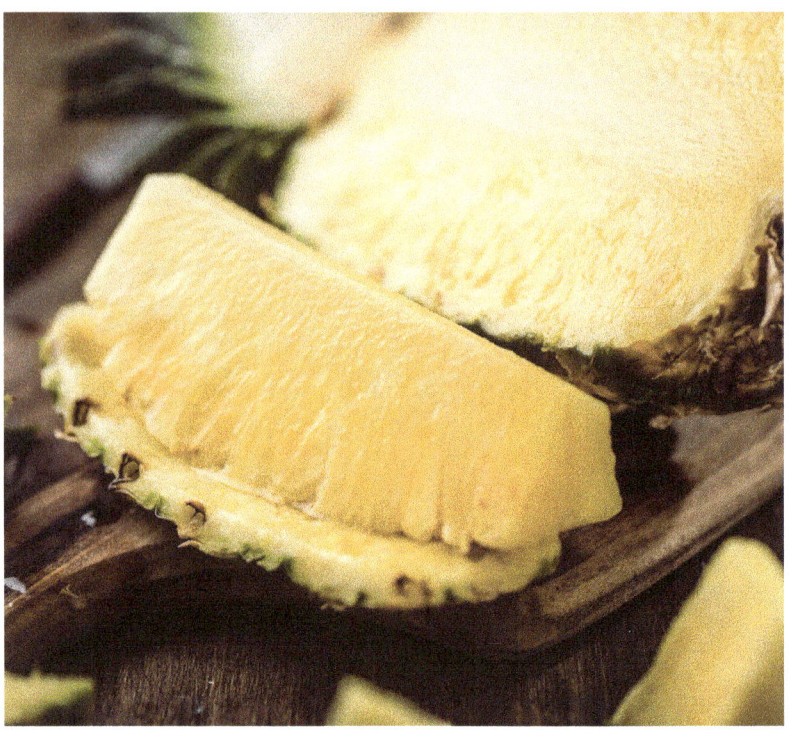

EAT FOR LONGEVITY

It took about 3 months of whole food, plant-based eating for all my cravings for sugar, fat, salt, fast food, and junk food to go away. Now, that stuff doesn't even look like food to me anymore. I stopped eating meat suddenly when it began to make me feel weepy and sad, and started tasting like suffering. Then, after learning about negative health effects of dairy, I gradually I cleared my fridge of eggs, butter, yogurt and cheeses. I was recovering from long Covid at the time and thought trying a fully whole foods, plant-based diet would help.

I've come off of the two blood pressure medicines I was on, lost some waistline inches, got my stamina and zest for life back, stopped experiencing chronic pain and almost never run out of energy anymore. I struggle sometimes and get sad like everyone does, but I mostly wake up happy, stay productive and creative all day long, and go to bed satisfied. My diet is a huge part of this.

My life changed when I read *How Not to Die: Discover the Foods Scientifically Proven to Prevent and Reverse Disease* by Dr. Michael Greger. It explores the most common disease-based causes of death in the United States, how to prevent and treat each one of them by using foods—and avoiding foods. Recent peer-reviewed scientific research studies appear on every page. I now cook from the *How Not to Die Cookbook* more than any other. There is a free website and email list with weekly nutrition videos, articles, and recipes at NutritionFacts.org.

Dr. Greger codified an ingredients list called "The Daily Dozen" (not to be confused with the dirty dozen!) The Daily Dozen describes the 12 categories we need to include in our diet every day for disease prevention and longevity:

- legumes
- whole grains
- greens
- cruciferous vegetables
- other vegetables
- berries
- other fruits
- flaxseeds
- other nuts and seeds
- herbs & spices
- beverages
- exercise

See the chart below for how many servings of each category to get every day. If you eat everything on the list, you will have the most nutrient-dense diet available on planet Earth. You'll get all the macronutrients (protein, fiber, carbohydrates) and all the micronutrients (vitamins, minerals, antioxidants) that you need, except for a few that require supplementation. You'll need to combine legumes and grains to give your body all 9 amino acids to form complete proteins. This can be within a 24-hour period, it doesn't need to be at every meal.

With the magical foods Mason jar life, it's easy to check off each of those categories every day. Even exercise is easy to check off with an evening walk, a daily constitutional to clear the head and lift the spirit after dinner. Take the air, my lovely friend.

Note: Vitamin Supplementation on a Plant-Based Diet

We used to get B-12 from bacteria in water, but now municipal tap water has chemicals that kill those good bugs. People on a plant-based diet must supplement their B-12 because serious nervous system damage can result from deficiency. A B-12 deficiency can cause anemia, blindness, and seizures, among other things. Vegans need 2500 mg. of B-12 per week, preferably in the form of cyanocobalamin rather than methylcobalamin (which does not absorb well). Many delicious vegan B-12 lozenges, sprays, gummies and tablets exist.

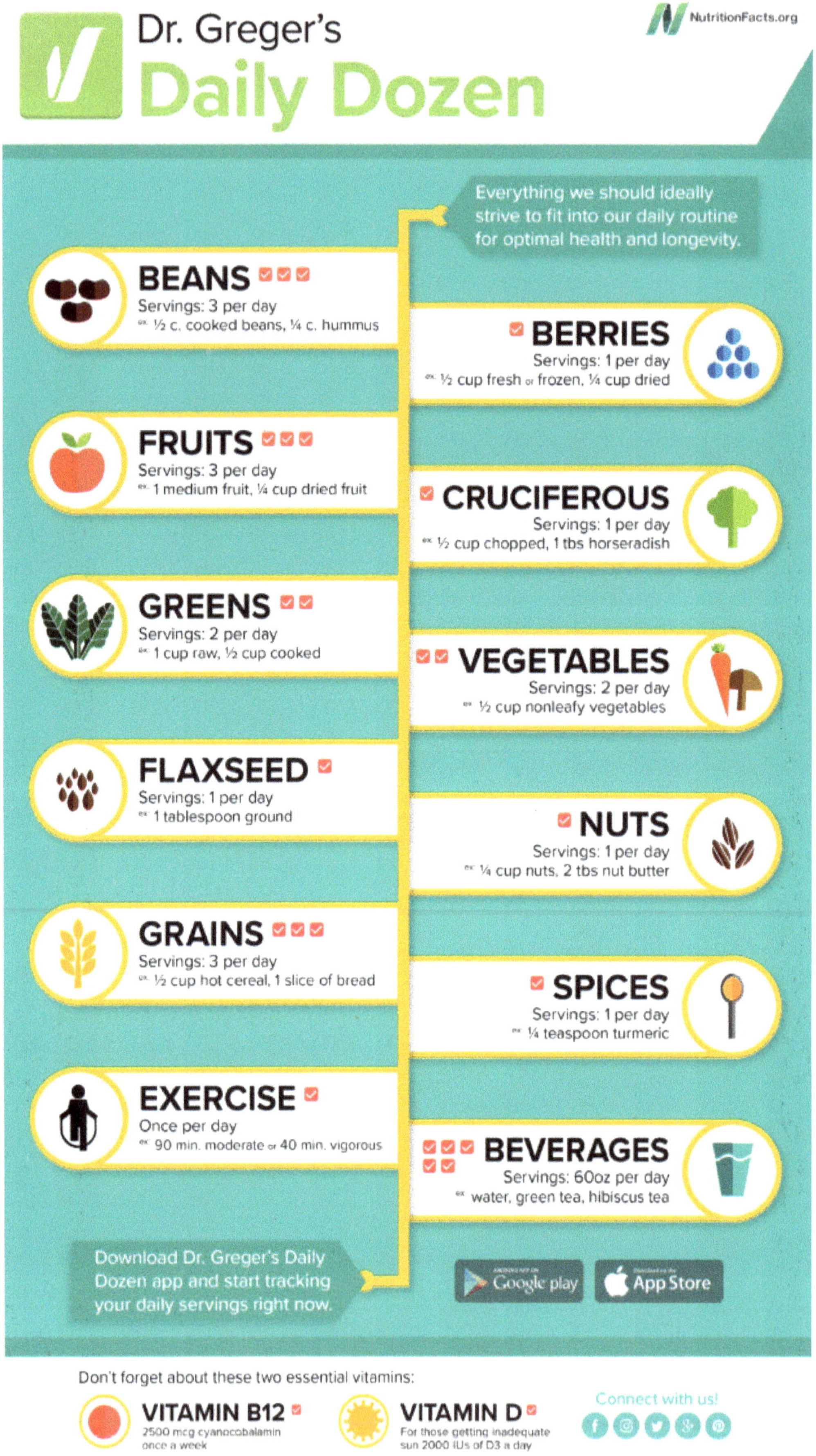

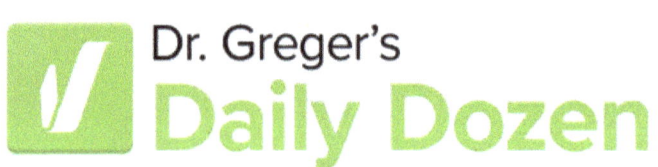 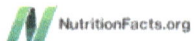

Dr. Greger's Daily Dozen

Everything we should ideally strive to fit into our daily routine for optimal health and longevity.

BEANS
Servings: 3 per day
ex ½ c. cooked beans, ¼ c. hummus

BERRIES
Servings: 1 per day
ex ½ cup fresh or frozen, ¼ cup dried

FRUITS
Servings: 3 per day
ex 1 medium fruit, ¼ cup dried fruit

CRUCIFEROUS
Servings: 1 per day
ex ½ cup chopped, 1 tbs horseradish

GREENS
Servings: 2 per day
ex 1 cup raw, ½ cup cooked

VEGETABLES
Servings: 2 per day
ex ½ cup nonleafy vegetables

FLAXSEED
Servings: 1 per day
ex 1 tablespoon ground

NUTS
Servings: 1 per day
ex ¼ cup nuts, 2 tbs nut butter

GRAINS
Servings: 3 per day
ex ½ cup hot cereal, 1 slice of bread

SPICES
Servings: 1 per day
ex ¼ teaspoon turmeric

EXERCISE
Once per day
ex 90 min. moderate or 40 min. vigorous

BEVERAGES
Servings: 60oz per day
ex water, green tea, hibiscus tea

Download Dr. Greger's Daily Dozen app and start tracking your daily servings right now.

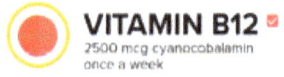 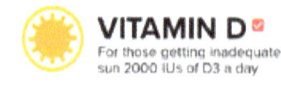

Don't forget about these two essential vitamins:

VITAMIN B12
2500 mcg cyanocobalamin once a week

VITAMIN D
For those getting inadequate sun 2000 IUs of D3 a day

Connect with us!

MAGICAL FOOD AND THE MASON JAR LIFE

How to Organize Your Refrigerator

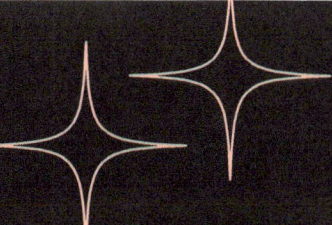

Everyone has their own preferences in fridge organization. Here's what works for me.

I organize the top shelf of the fridge left to right by meal. Soymilk, teas and breakfast jars are on the left of the top shelf, lunch pasta dishes and raw salads are stacked in the middle, and dinner soup and grains are on the top right. As I go through the day, I move through the top shelf of the fridge as if I'm reading a book, left to right.

I use the middle shelf for glass containers of raw veggies for snacking, dips, and any extra ready-to-eat foods such as hummus or defrosted meals from the freezer. Olives, applesauce, jars of pickled vegetables and other cold snack foods go here, as do peanut and almond butter. Anything ready-to-eat is visible and prominent at the very front of the shelf, and foods that keep longer or I eat less often are shelved behind that layer.

I use the bottom shelf for uncut raw vegetables and fruits in clear plastic boxes, and for breads, tortillas, bagels, etc. If I put fresh uncut produce in the fridge drawers, I'll forget about it and it will go bad. So I keep it visible at the front of the bottom shelf, with breads. The fridge drawers store bottled drinks and vitamins and supplements.

In one layer at the back of the top shelf, I also keep the things I use most often when cooking: miso paste, vegetable broth, bouillon paste and jarred sauces, easy to grab.

The door of the fridge holds vegan butter, jams and marmalades, lemon and lime juice, ketchup, sauces, salad dressing and other small, bottled goods.

Looking at my refrigerator makes me feel calm and organized. I know exactly where everything is, and there's no clutter or disorder. Everything has a use and a place. It will fall into disorder at times, of course; chaos is natural. Then it beckons me back to tend it, wipe down the shelves, simplify and honor it with care, putting the contents into order.

How to Organize Your Freezer

My freezer used to be crammed with processed foods like ice cream, egg rolls, French fries, fake meats and frozen dinners. It was a cacophony of colored boxes and I felt like a rabid raccoon when I dug through it. When I decided to move to a whole food, plant-based diet, I gave all that food away. Now my freezer has ample space for a rotating cast of beans, veggies, fruits, and home-cooked leftovers.

It can benefit your health and bank account to use your freezer primarily for frozen fruits, veggies, and cooked beans. Frozen produce is an efficient choice at the store because it's already been washed, peeled, and chopped for you–and is frozen at peak freshness, preserving more of its nutrients. Beans are easy to pressure cook and save in gallon bags for use in smoothies and recipes. These ingredients are cleaner and less expensive than processed food.

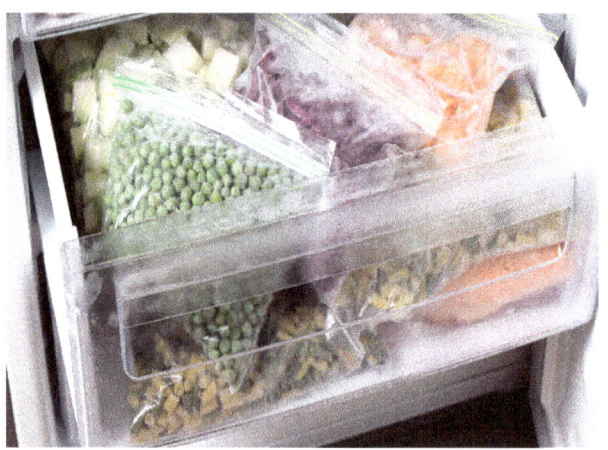

Like the fridge, I organize the freezer by meal. The top section is breakfast (large bags of frozen fruit and chopped leafy greens for smoothies.) The middle section is lunch and dinner ingredients (chopped vegetables, cooked beans, faux chik'n patties, vegetable broth.) The bottom section is frozen meals that I've prepped and cooked earlier, labeled, and stored in square containers that I can just reach in and grab, then microwave and eat.

Here's what I keep in the freezer:

- Bananas, peeled for smoothies
  (3-4 fresh bunches fills a gallon-sized Ziploc bag)
- Berries like blueberries, raspberries, and strawberries for smoothies (I buy a 3-lb frozen bag)
- Frozen chopped leafy greens like collards and kale for smoothies (I buy 2 pounds of each and fill two gallon-sized Ziploc bags)
- Red grapes for snacking (the most delectable summertime frozen treat)
- Frozen faux chik'n patties and nuggets for visiting children
- Frozen broccoli, cauliflower, green peas, and edamame
- Frozen, cubed yams and butternut squash
- Pressure-cooked beans in gallon Ziploc bags with flat bottoms
- Homemade veggie broth
- Homemade fruit popsicles
- Serving-portion size meals labeled with date and contents

How to Keep a Food Inventory

Keeping a food inventory helps make sure that all the food in the fridge gets eaten, and the bulk goods are used in great variety.

I handwrite the inventory weekly on a grocery list pad that goes on the fridge door. It looks a bit like this. I consult it like a menu at a restaurant.

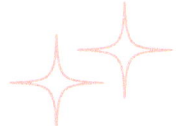

READY-TO-EAT	*FRESH/RAW*	*FROZEN*
pesto pasta	yams	smoothie fruit
ginger coleslaw	beets & beet greens	veggie dumplings
broccoli cheeze soup	avocados	red beans and rice
baked apples	arugula	fire-roasted veggies
pumpkin tofu pudding	tofu	kale & collards
overnight oats	carrots	chickpeas & navy beans
cut cantaloupe	cauliflower	popsicles
hibiscus tea	broccoli sprouts	peanut yam soup
pickled carrots	onions, garlic & ginger	butternut squash
peanut & almond butter		green peas
hummus		broccoli
soymilk		grapes

How To Stay Happy And Avoid Eating Junk

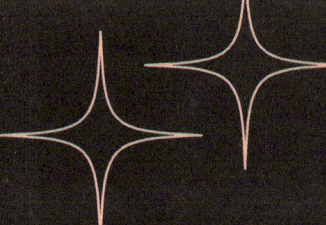

We can all be tempted by bad-for-us foods. I have a cute trash panda inside me like everyone else, of course! I have to use mind tricks to avoid fake food and unhealthy choices so I can stay committed to my body and budget. When I feel scared or upset, I have impulses to eat salty, sweet and greasy food. When I query my tongue, I can usually identify the flavor desire and figure out a work-around, how to meet the desire in a whole food, plant-based way.

Identify the Flavor Desire and Find a Healthy Substitution

- If I find myself craving fast food French fries, I identify that the real flavor desire is salt. I'll have some crunchy veggies dipped in soy sauce, or some seasoned dry shiitake mushrooms.
- If I crave ice cream, I know it is cold and sweet I really want. I'll have frozen grapes.
- If I crave cheese, it is melty texture and fat I want. I'll make warm, melted cashew queso (p. 83) and dip carrots or corn chips into it.
- If I want tart candy, it is acid my body is signaling for, so I'll drink a glass of water with a splash of apple cider vinegar, lemon juice and maple syrup, or eat a sour-sweet fruit like dried cherries.
- If I hanker for something fiery like Hot Cheetos, a couple of pieces of candied ginger root do the trick, or some wasabi powder on raw peanuts.

And of course, it's not the worst thing in the world to fall off the wagon or have a wallow in the grease. It's progress we're going for, not perfection.

DEFYING FAST FOOD URGES TAKES EFFORT

I also use mental imagery to keep myself from patronizing fast food joints. When stressed, I feel drawn to McDonald's French fries, Popeye's biscuits, Sonic tater tots and grilled cheese, and other salt-drenched comforts. My inner child still thinks those places are where you go for a birthday party or when you get a good report card.

But eating fast food isn't in line with my values in any way–from their environmental destruction to vast animal cruelty to exploitative labor practices. I may feel temporarily satisfied, but then I have a moral hangover and don't feel great about my choices.

MAGICAL FOOD AND THE MASON JAR LIFE

Now, when I crave it, I start by imagining eating the fast-food meal after it has sat out for a day–by which time it's hard as a rock and tasteless, an inanimate object.
I then take it a step further and start imagining that I have to eat the sign. Yes, I have to eat the logo and the sign. When I'm drawn to turn my car into the drive-through line, I have to mentally bite into the large plastic yellow arches of McDonalds and imagine chewing and swallowing it, my stomach filling up with the pieces. It isn't appetizing. This usually cures the draw.

What mental imagery helps you keep on track with the things you do and don't want to experience?

EATING FOOD ALIGNED WITH OUR VALUES CREATES HAPPINESS

Everyone finds what works best for them and their own body, in their own time.

In 2022, I read an article in the New York Times that had a quiz for readers about the most important actions a single individual can take to slow climate change and reduce their own carbon dioxide emissions. I failed the quiz, like most readers. I learned that adopting a mostly plant-based diet is the single most effective thing anyone can do to avert climate catastrophe–more than recycling, composting, driving an electric car, reducing flights, and many other actions.

I thought, *I can do that. That's a no-brainer. Yes. Today. I'm on it.* Grief and fear I feel over global warming, species loss and our hurting earth has eased some, because I know I'm doing what I can, in my small way. This gives me hope. Taking an action shifts the feeling state, the field in which our perception and meaning is generated. It opens up possibility. That's a key to happiness.

But acting with intention over and over is not easy, especially when you are accustomed to eating differently. I often wanted to eat fish and had to use mental imagery to shift that desire.

I got this idea from Jonathan Safran Froer's book *Eating Animals*. When I want to eat a fish filet, I try to imagine the "bycatch" also on the table–the other fish, dolphins, seals, sharks, stingrays, turtles, seabirds and ocean creatures that are caught, killed and discarded by the nets of industrial fishing operations. These nets are 50 to 80 miles long. Imagining that size brings tears to my eyes.

For every one pound of fish on the plate, up to six pounds of other fish and ocean creatures are killed and discarded. So, I can't plan to sit down to eat one piece of fish without visualizing all the other dead fish piled up on the table and thanking them as well. Then I see clearly that the cost is too great. I don't want to kill all these living creatures just to eat one. (Factory fish farming is really no better.)

Regarding factory farming of animals, I've chosen just one visual detail from each of the animal's lives in these settings to bring to mind when I am tempted to have a burger or chocolate milk. The memory cue works to end my interest in eating that animal product. I make an exception for dairy products from animals I have met on humane farms I have seen. I do this while remembering that we must immediately phase out animal agriculture altogether, globally, to have a fighting chance at slowing climate change.

This helps me keep my choices aligned with my values—which contributes to happiness. And the happier I am, the more readily I can access my own magic. Perhaps the same is true for you.

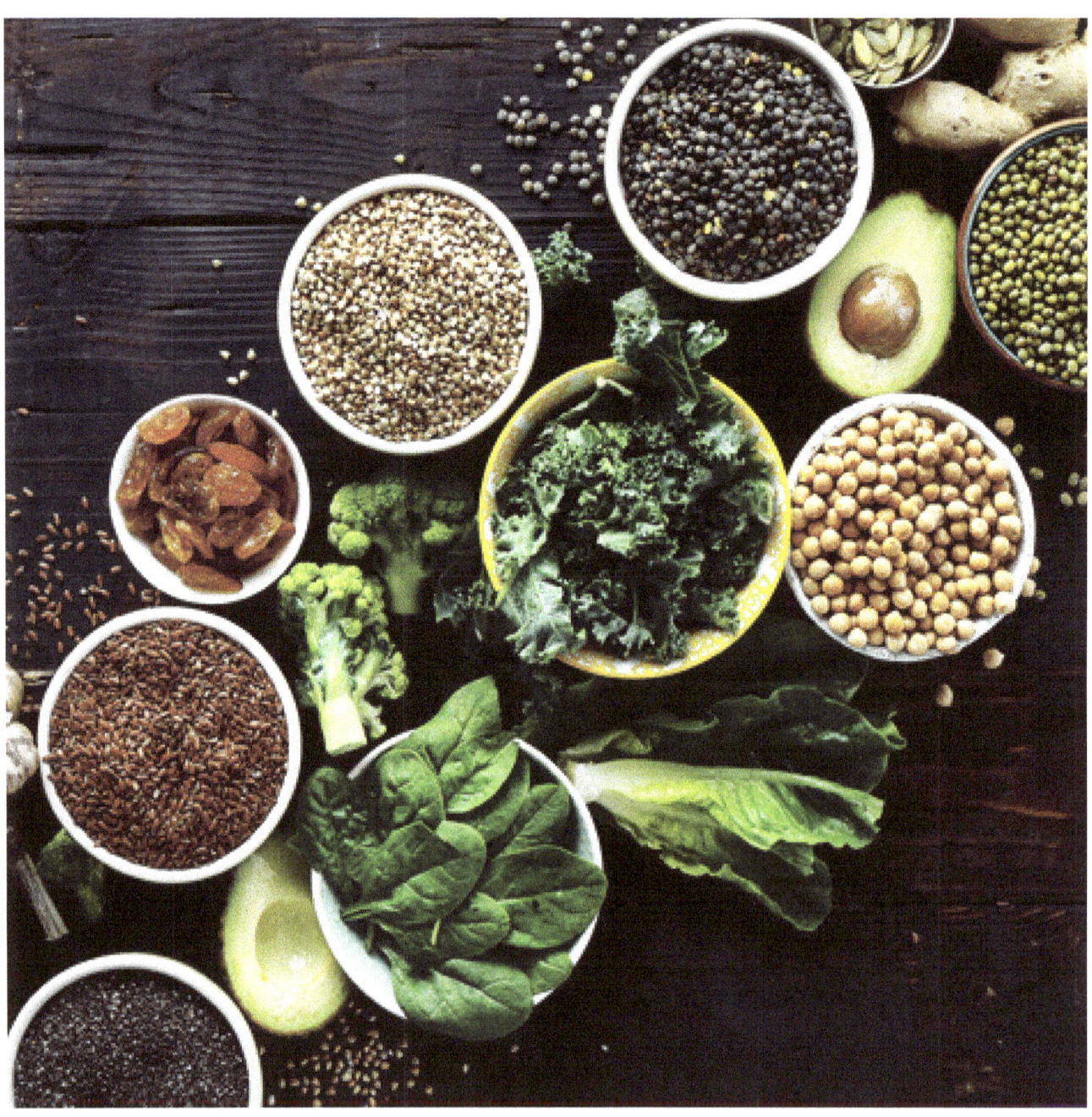

MAGICAL FOOD AND THE MASON JAR LIFE

Food and Water Storage for Emergencies

Things are getting more unpredictable around here! When a natural disaster or other emergency happens, you'll be glad to have thought ahead about your basic needs and those of your loved ones and neighbors.

My mother calls her bulk goods jars her "apocalypse pantry." When Hurricane Ida knocked out the electricity to New Orleans for weeks, she lived just fine on canned food and bulk goods. She has enough to survive for three months.

Hurricane Katrina and subsequent disasters have shown us that we cannot rely on government, cities, or FEMA to take care of our basic needs. We must be prepared to take care of ourselves and our neighbors, especially children and those who are disabled or elderly. Whether that is helping everyone to evacuate or sheltering in place and cooking a huge pot of beans and rice for the block, it's up to us to be the heroes we need. Neighbors rescued neighbors in flooded New Orleans for many days before any officials arrived on the scene to help. Dogs swimming in floodwaters tried to save people before the National Guard did.

Caring for ourselves and our neighbors includes making sure we have enough food, water, medicine and fuel stored.

If a severe weather event is on the way, put as much water as possible into jars, buckets, plugged bathtubs, etc. I keep ten collapsible water storage cubes so I can have 50 gallons of water in case of emergency.

Each adult needs half a gallon to drink per day, plus water for cooking, bathing, and toilet flushing. It takes 1-3 gallons to flush a toilet and 2 gallons to wash dishes in a two-bucket system (one bucket for soapy water and scrubbing, one bucket to rinse). If the tap water is broken for a week to ten days, having 50 gallons on hand will keep a small household functioning.

Calculate the amount of dry bulk food you'll need for two weeks to feed yourself and others 2000 calories a day using a [food storage calculator](#). You'll need to combine legumes and grains to give your body all 9 amino acids to form complete proteins. This can be within a 24-hour period, it doesn't need to be at every meal. I recommend every household have at least 20 pounds of dry beans and 20 pounds of dry grains per person stored (including quinoa, which is a complete protein by itself).

Plan how you'll cook if the electricity and/or gas is no longer working. I have a small charcoal barbecue and a 2-burner propane campstove with spare propane stored in the garage. If that runs out, I can cook over a wood fire with a cast iron grate for pans and a tripod for hanging a cast iron pot.

I could also use an electric converter outlet in my car's cigarette lighter jack for power, as long as I have gasoline. During Winter Storm Uri that knocked out power for a week in Texas during sub-freezing temperatures and iced over streets, I discovered that a car cigarette jack converter with a 3-prong outlet can power a pressure cooker.

In that disaster, the water pipes froze and broke all over town. We had to melt snow for drinking since I had not stored water. It was an eye-opening two weeks before the pipes were repaired and the water worked again. I learned my lesson!

When a natural disaster takes place again, I hope to be better prepared. I've stored 25-lbs each of red lentils, garbanzo beans, soybeans, quinoa, oats, brown rice and dried fruit, as well as canned goods, dried fruit, oil, sugar, B-12, prescription medications, sprouting seeds and spices. This is an investment meant to provide three months of food for two adults. I hope it never needs to be used.

Even if you can't make such an investment, or even get food from a food pantry, you can slowly sock away a long-term food storage tub over time. Whatever your circumstances, take care of yourself and think ahead to how much food and water you'll need in an emergency for yourself and your loved ones.

Now that we've discussed all eventualities, let's get on to favorite recipes!

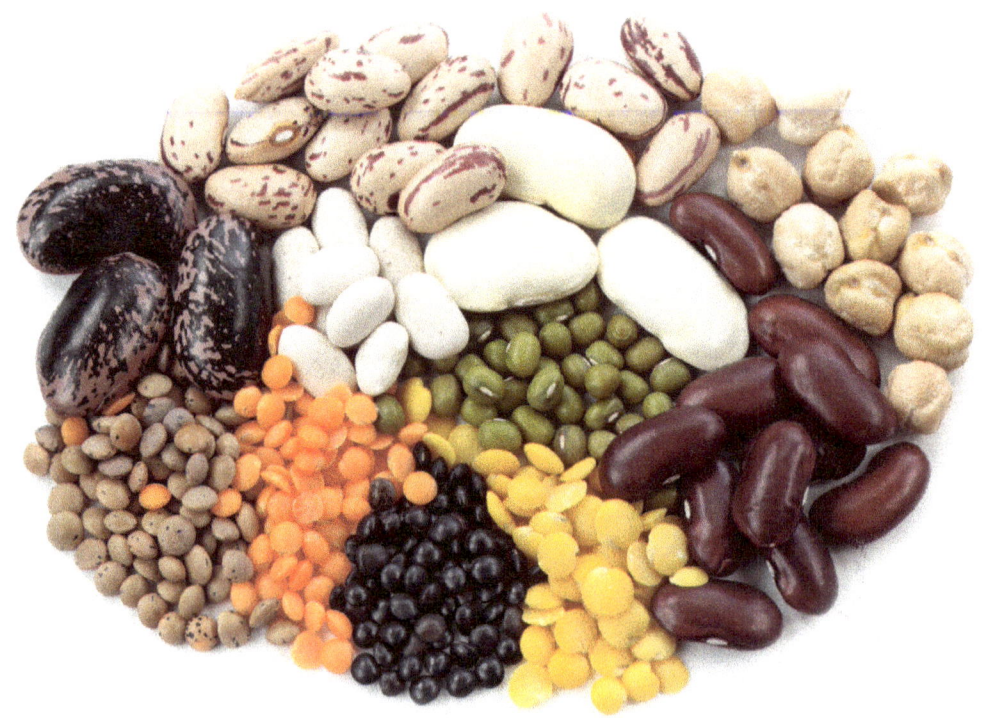

MAGICAL FOOD AND THE MASON JAR LIFE

Recipes

I'm not a trained chef; I'm a home cook. I've never taken a cooking class except at my mother's knee. I put together this collection of recipes by culling what I cook most often from my binder of handwritten recipe cards, splashed and stained and scribbled with notes.

The recipes here are ones I learned from friends and relatives and adapted from various cookbooks with my own substitutions. I've made each of these recipes scores of times, but I'm sure you can improve upon them and match your own tastes. Please take them and make them your own—and let me know how they turn out!

Blessings on your food, your hands, your table and your people.

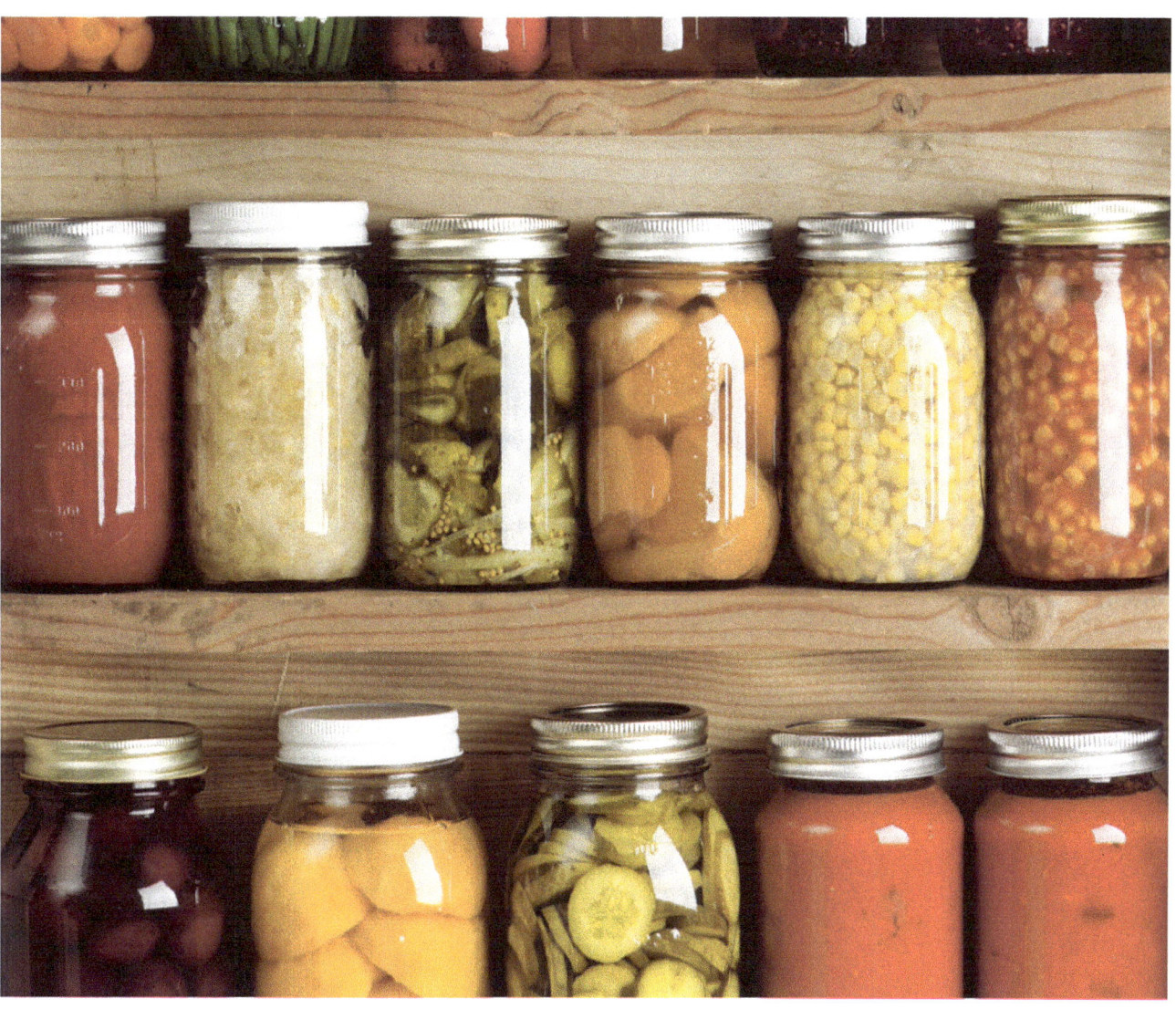

Plant-Based Milks

Makes 1/2 gallon (64 oz), or 8 cups

- 1 cup dry beans or nuts, soaked overnight in 4 cups filtered water
- 8 cups filtered water
- 1 teaspoon cinnamon, *optional*
- 1 teaspoon vanilla extract, *optional*
- 1/4 teaspoon salt
- 1 teaspoon powdered calcium citrate if desired for calcium supplementation, *optional*

SOYMILK

Making plant-based milk with beans that require cooking, such as soymilk, can be done on the stove with a large pot, a blender and a cheesecloth for straining. People have done this for centuries. However, it takes a lot of effort and time. If you invest in a plant-based milk maker, making your soymilk becomes easy and fast.

A plant-based milk maker looks like an electric kettle from the outside. I like the Soyabella Plant-Based Milk Maker and use it at least weekly. The Soyabella is an all-in-one machine to cook and grind your raw ingredients, making frothy, delicious milks. Inside the carafe, it has a filter basket and a blade. You fill the basket with 1/2 of your soaked soybeans and fill the carafe with fresh water.

On the hot cook cycle, the machine boils the water and cooks the soaked soybeans, then grinds them with the blade and forces the water through the filter basket. In about half an hour, 32 ounces of hot, frothy milk is made.

Wait 15 minutes for the machine and milk to cool, then remove the filter basket from the motor head and blade using the included drip cup. Pour the soymilk into your large Mason jar, using a small strainer over the mouth of the jar to catch foam and pulp. Add vanilla, salt and cinnamon, and you have a heavenly high-protein beverage.

It's important to quickly dump, rinse and scrub the filter basket so the fine stainless steel mesh doesn't get clogged. I scrub with a rough abrasive scrubber and a toothbrush for about 3 minutes under running water each time I use it.

I consume a half-gallon of soymilk each week, so I run two cycles. After the first jug of soymilk is made, I immediately refill the carafe with water and the filter basket with soaked soybeans and run another cycle.

The pulp left over from soybeans is called okara and is highly nutritious (if a bit grainy). It can be used in baking and soups, or as a nitrogen-adding compost. The pulp left over from making nutmilks is also excellent fiber to use in baking.

OAT MILK, ALMOND MILK, CASHEW MILK

A vegan milk maker will also make wonderful raw oat and nut milks (which require no cooking) by grinding, mixing and straining them for you, without heating the water.

Making cold or raw milks, such as nut milk or oat milk, can also be done easily without a vegan milk machine. Add 2 cup of oats or nuts to six cups water in a high-speed blender, and blend till the solids are liquid. Then, pour the results through a cheesecloth or fine mesh strainer, squeezing the cheesecloth or pressing the ingredients through the strainer with the back of a large spoon to extract all the milk. It will be delicious. Adjust the proportions to your liking.

SUPPLEMENTING WITH CALCIUM

Most packaged plant milks in stores have added calcium to make them more nutritionally comparable to cow's milk. It is easy to add calcium to your plant-based milks, if you like. Just buy powdered calcium citrate and put two teaspoons in your 64-oz jar of plant milk. Shake the closed jar before you pour from it to get the calcium into suspension.

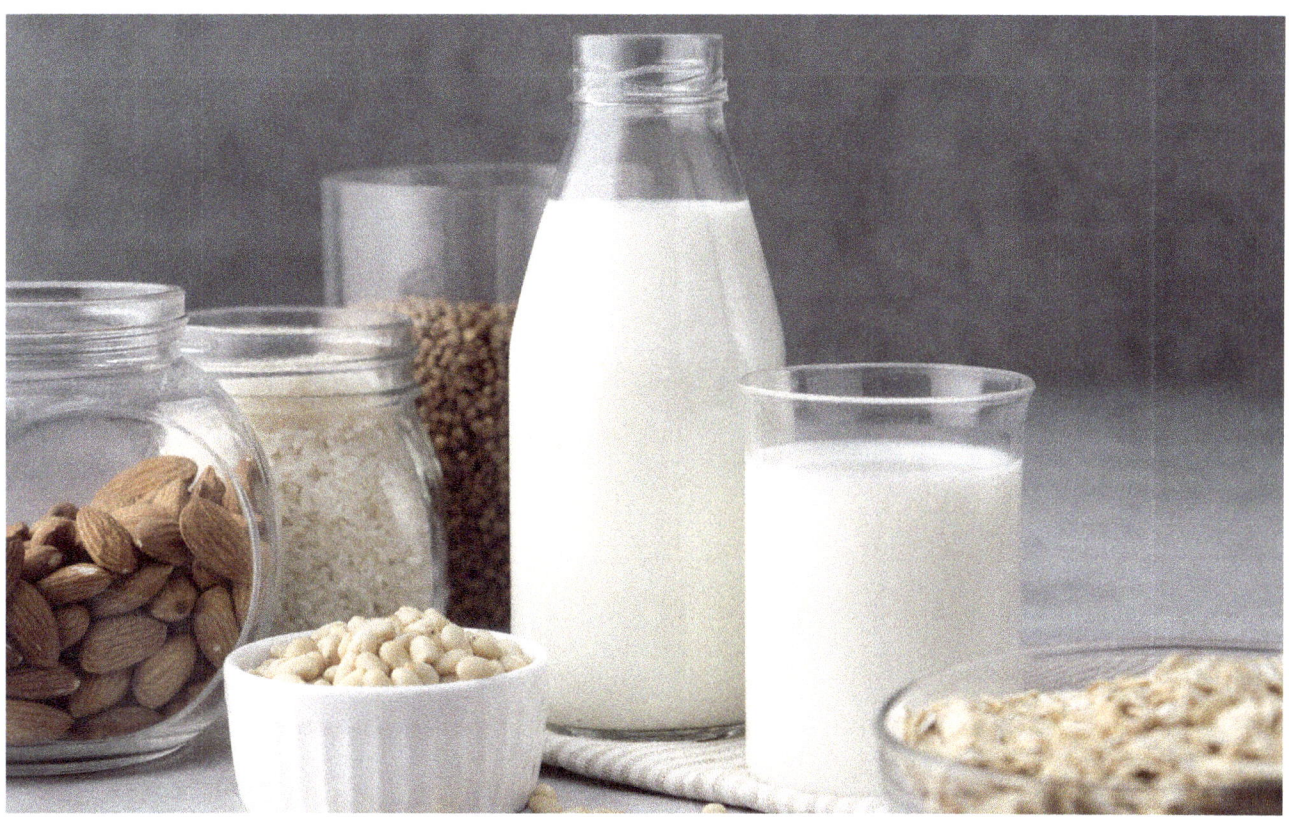

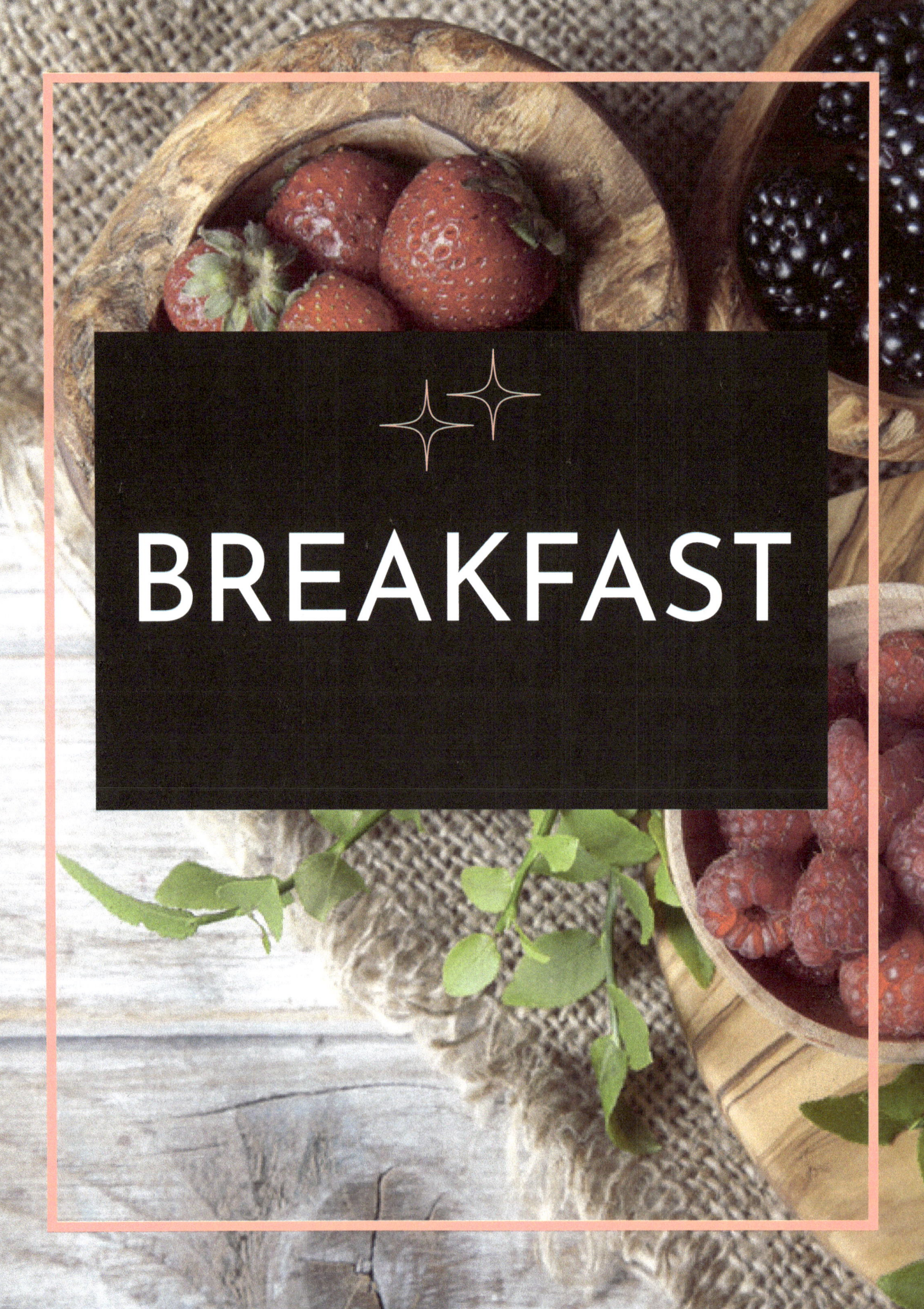

BREAKFAST

Overnight Oats

3/4 cup rolled or steel-cut oats

1 Tablespoon chia seeds

handful of blueberries

plant milk to cover the oats, with an extra inch

splash of maple syrup

dash of vanilla

1/2 teaspoon cinnamon

INSTRUCTIONS

1) In a pint Mason jar, add all of the ingredients listed above.

2) Stir it all together and put it in the fridge. Heat it in the morning if you prefer, with 30-60 seconds in the microwave. Add more plant milk if desired.

A jar starts the day off right and will keep you full till lunchtime.

Note: This recipe won't work with instant oats–they need to be rolled oats or steel-cut oats to hold their shape.

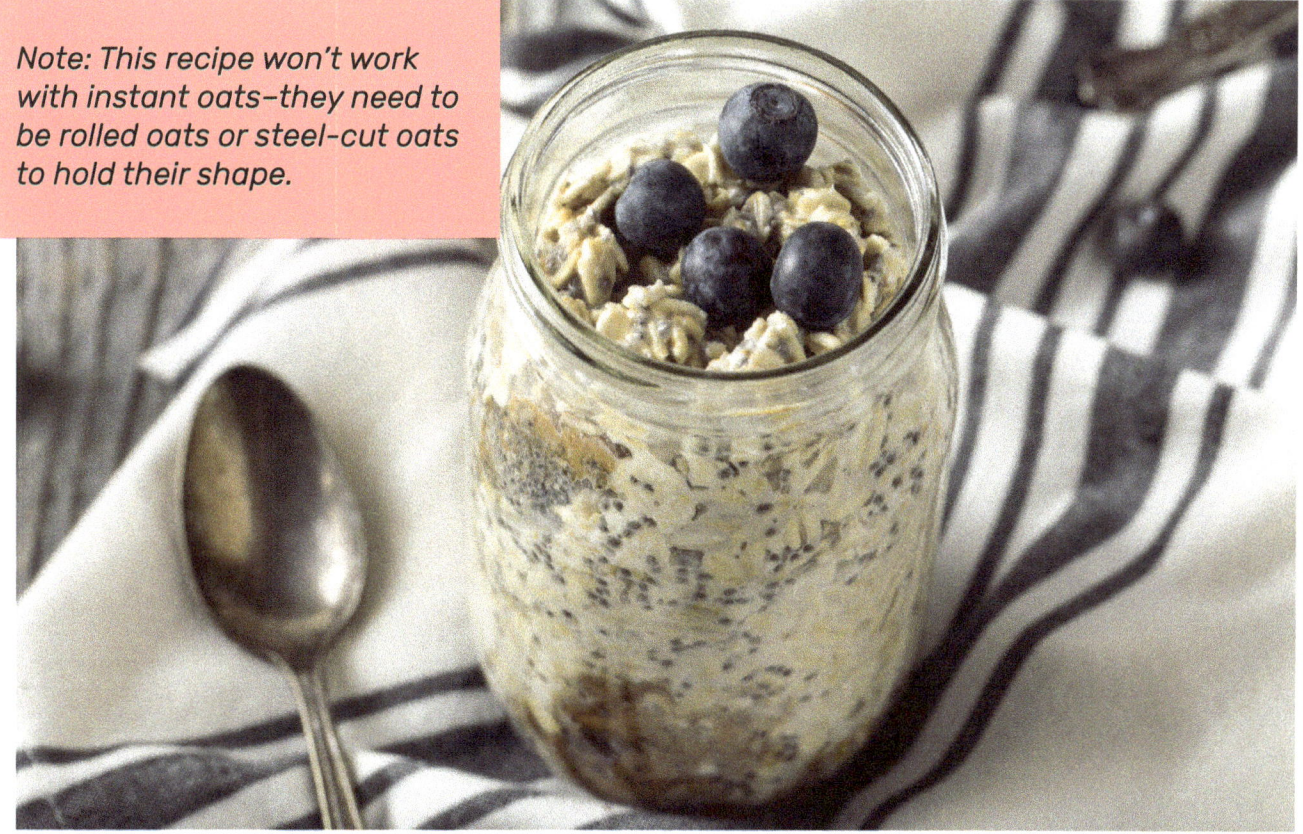

Luxurious Chia Pudding

Servings: 2-4

You really only need three ingredients for this: chia seeds, non-dairy milk, and a sweetener. Add berries and a dash of vanilla and salt to perfect it. Add any toppings you like to boost the flavor. It's loaded with protein, fiber and Omega-3s.

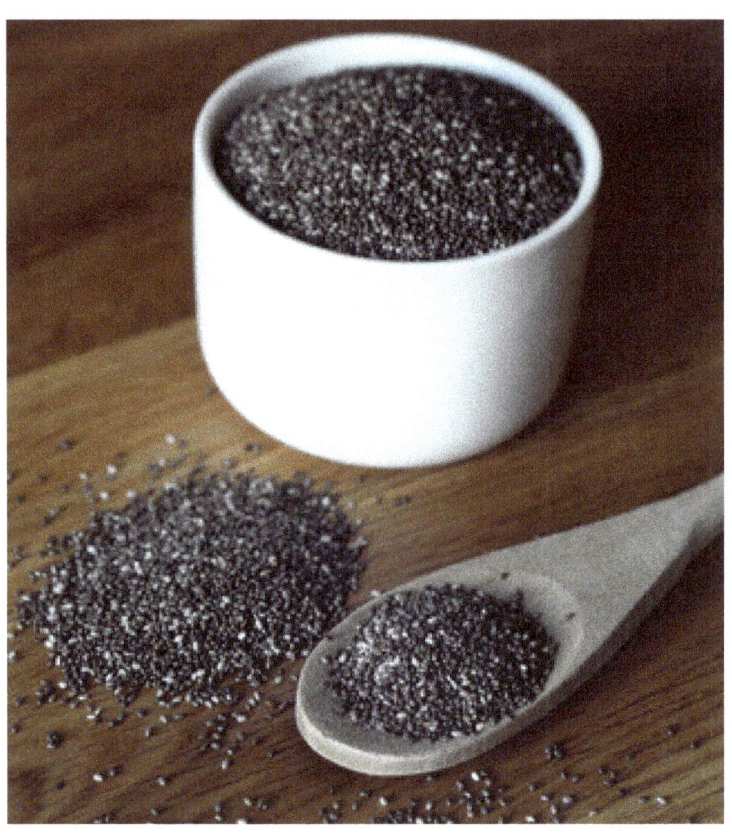

3 Tablespoons chia seeds

1 cup plant milk of your choice

a splash of maple syrup to taste

dash of vanilla

pinch of salt

berries or any sliced fresh fruit

INSTRUCTIONS

1) Add half the ingredients to one pint (16 oz.) jar and half the ingredients to another pint jar, as the chia seeds will swell. Mix well.

Pumpkin Tofu Pudding

Servings: 2-4

This smooth, creamy dish tastes like pumpkin pie in a jar—and it's extremely nutritious and filling.

- 1 block tofu (any kind of tofu works; silken soft tofu will be the creamiest)
- 1 can packed pumpkin or sweet potato
- 1/8 cup to 1/4 cup plant-based milk or water, as preferred
- 1 to 2 Tablespoons sugar, maple syrup, honey, or stevia, to taste
- 1 teaspoon cinnamon
- 1/2 teaspoon allspice
- 1/4 teaspoon clove
- 1/4 teaspoon nutmeg
- 1/4 teaspoon cardamom
- dash of vanilla

INSTRUCTIONS

1) Add all ingredients to a high-speed blender and blend until the texture is delicate and creamy. Adjust spices and sweetener to taste.

2) Fills two pint jars, which can be two or four servings, as you wish.

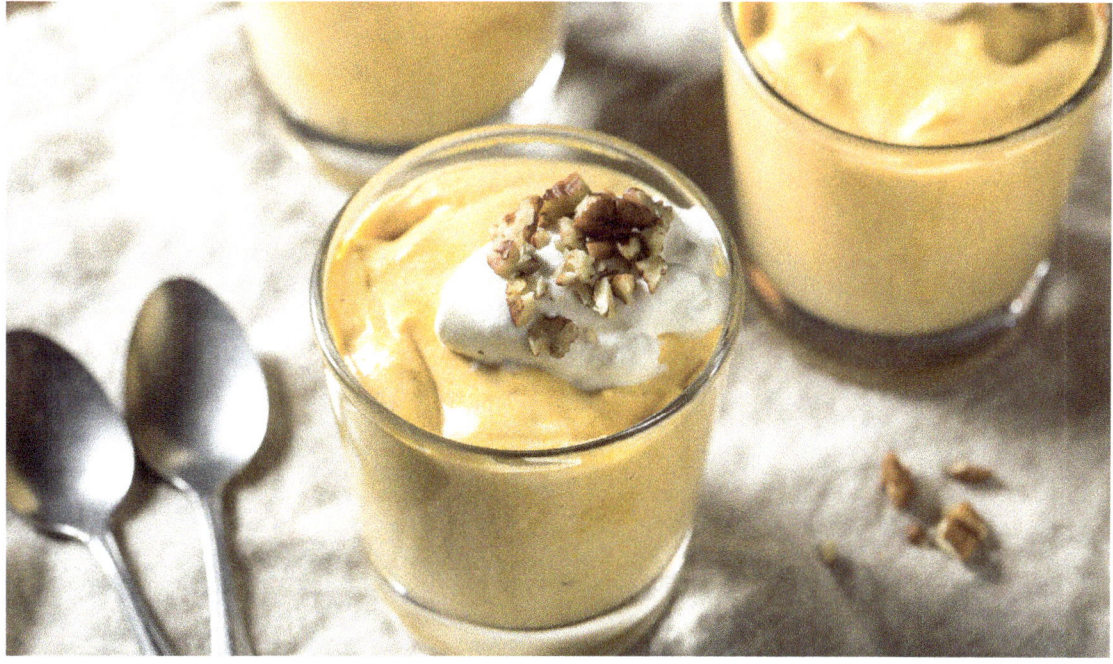

Choose-Your-Own-Adventure Smoothie

Servings: 2

With basic smoothie proportions, you can make your smoothie recipes out of whatever fruits, veggies, nuts/nut butter and liquid you have on hand.

If you value extra protein, add a lightly sweetened protein powder, soymilk, cooked unseasoned beans, or tofu. If you like it creamier, use a plant-based milk or add some raw rolled oats. If you like it sweeter, add fruit juice, stevia or even a dollop of maple syrup.

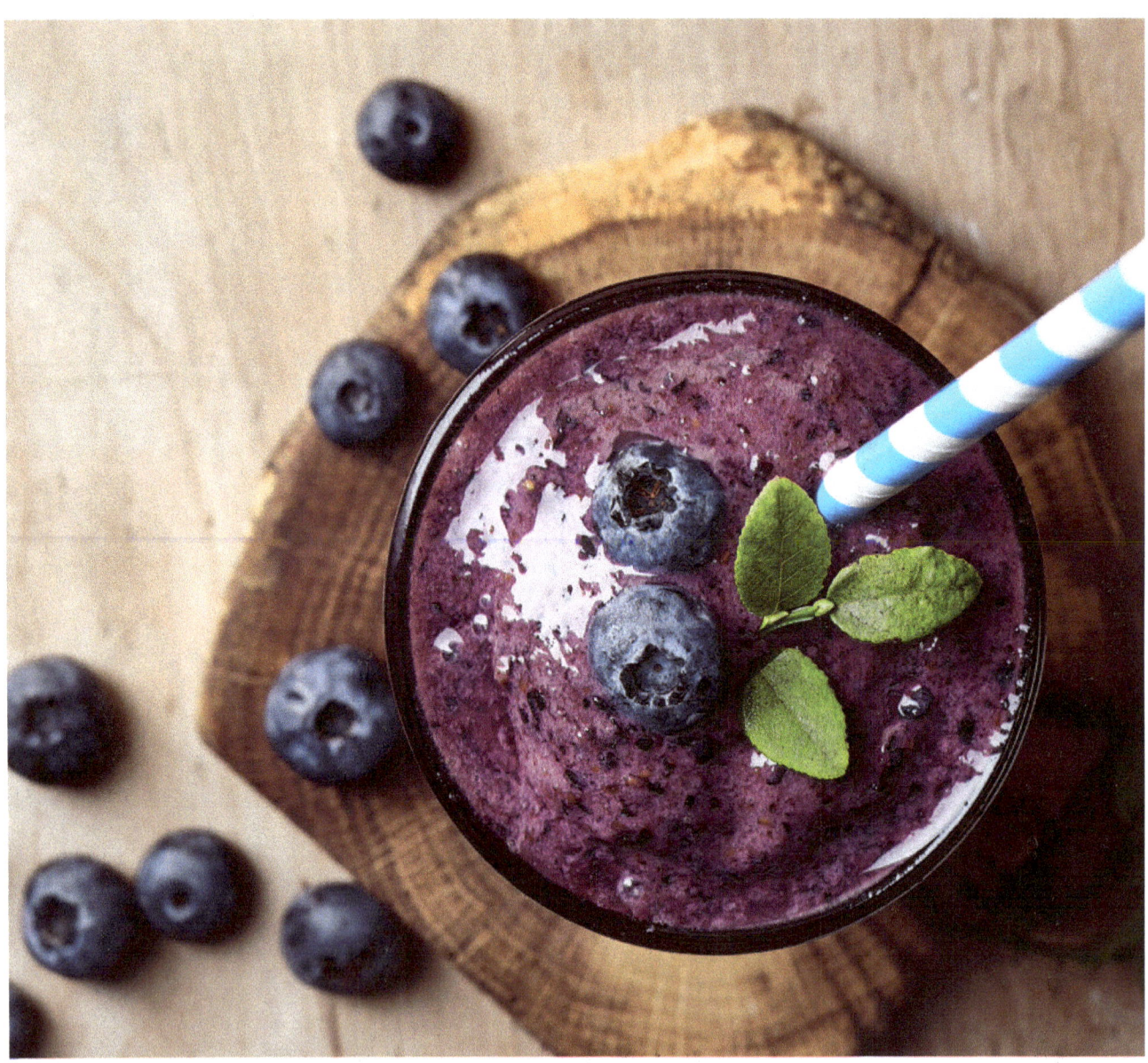

Choose-Your-Own-Adventure Smoothie Cont'd

① ADD FRUIT (FRESH OR FROZEN)

Always:
1/2 to 1 banana to make it creamy

Extra Options:
apricot, apple, avocado, berries, citrus, cucumber, dates, grapes, kiwi, lime, mango, melon, papaya, peach, pear, pineapple

② ADD GREENS

Always:
Up to 1 cup fresh or frozen leafy greens, or up to 50% of smoothie

Extra Options:
arugula, basil, beet greens, collard greens, herbs, kale, leftover salad greens, lettuce, mustard greens, parsley, Romaine lettuce, spinach, Swiss chard, turnip greens

③ ADD NUTS/SEEDS/NUT BUTTERS

Always:
1 T ground flax seeds, because it has 100X more powerhouse cancer-preventing lignans than any other nut/seed.

Extra Options:
almonds/almond butter, Brazil nuts, cashews, chia seeds, hazelnuts, hemp hearts, pecans, peanuts/peanut butter, sesame seeds, sunflower seeds/sunbutter, tahini/sesame butter, walnuts

④ ADD LIQUID

Always:
1/2 to 2 cups water or ice

Extra Options:
coconut water, coffee, fruit juice, plant-based milk (oat milk, rice milk, soymilk, etc.), tea

⑤ ADD PROTEIN

Orgain Organic Vanilla or Chocolate Protein Powder (sweetened with stevia), Garden of Life Organic Vegan Vanilla or Chocolate Protein Powder (sweetened with stevia), Nutriva Organic Hemp Protein Powder (unsweetened), raw tofu or soymilk, cooked white beans, black beans or chickpeas

⑥ BLEND, TASTE, THEN SWEETEN IF NEEDED

Optional:
agave nectar, blackstrap molasses (full of iron!), brown rice syrup, dates, honey, fruit juice, maple syrup, stevia, sugar (brown or turbinado)

BREAKFAST

Choose-Your-Own-Adventure Smoothie Cont'd

OTHER SMOOTHIE INGREDIENTS

Many other vegetables are great in smoothies. When veggies start to get tired in my fridge, or I've had them for too many meals, I throw them in a smoothie and adjust the other ingredients to make it taste good. If the smoothie is veggie-forward, add sweetened protein powder, pitted dates or another sweetener.

Additional Options:
- cabbage, cooked
- carrots, cooked
- celery
- ginger root
- oatmeal, raw or cooked
- lentils, cooked
- squash, cooked
- turmeric root
- whole grains, cooked
- yams, cooked
- zucchini, raw or cooked

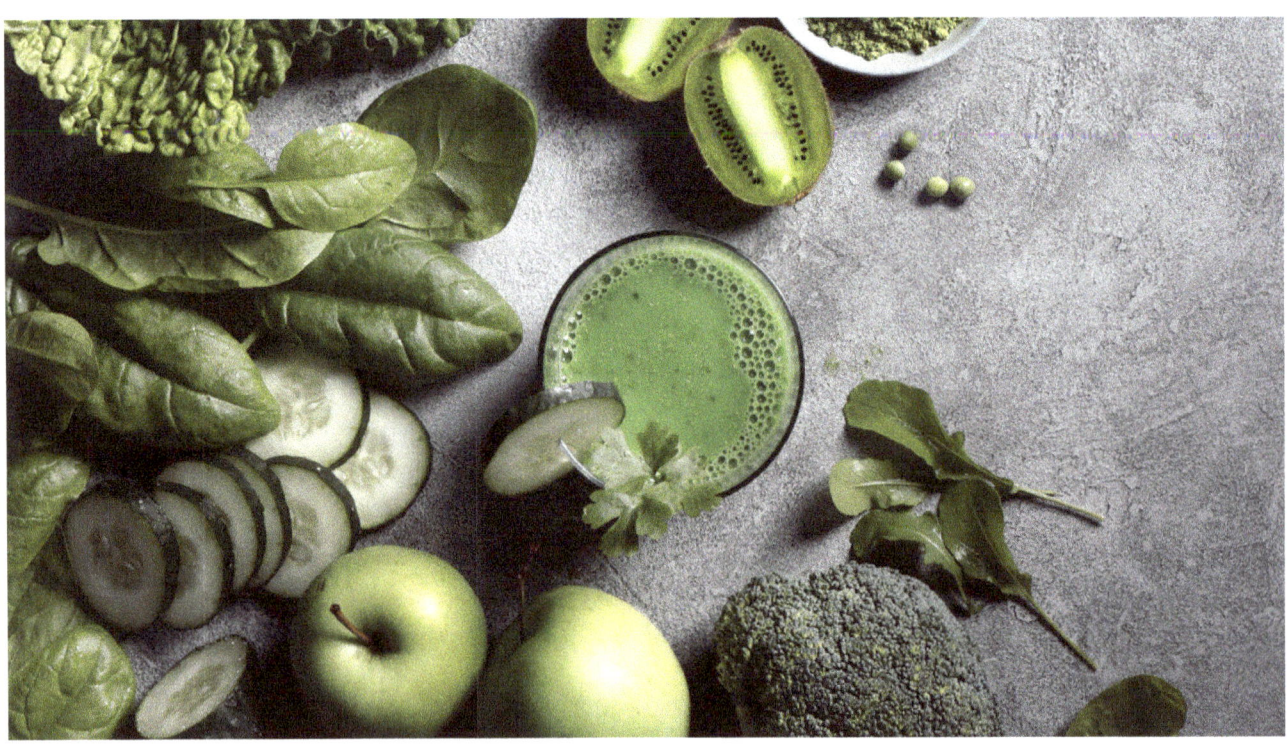

Berry Green Smoothie

This is my daily smoothie. I prep 3 ahead in the fridge and drink half a smoothie every day. I love to get leafy cruciferous greens like collards or kale in the morning. I can feel my body crying out for the greens if I miss it!

- 1 cup chopped frozen chopped greens or the equivalent fresh (such as 1 large collard greens leaf stripped off the spine, or 1 cup spinach or baby kale)
- 1/2 to 1 whole banana, to taste
- A nice handful of blueberries (around 1/3 cup)
- 2 Tablespoons ground flax seeds
- 1/4 cup vanilla protein powder, *optional* (use a powder with a little sweetness to counteract the greens—or add two dates)
- 1/2 cup to 2 cups water, to taste (or sub 1 cup soymilk for more protein)
- 1 Tablespoon of broccoli sprouts to keep the cancer away, *optional*

INSTRUCTIONS

1) To meal prep these, add ingredients for smoothies that you will blend in the mornings to the jar of a bullet blender and keep your prepped jars in the fridge. If you don't have a bullet blender, use a quart Mason jar or Ziploc bag to hold the ingredients that you'll pour into a regular blender. You can even prep a dozen smoothies in advance if you add the fruit and greens to quart Ziplock bags and keep them in the freezer—adding liquid, protein and nuts/seeds when it's time to eat.

2) Blend smoothie for 45 seconds or until smooth.

Peach Pie Smoothie

Servings: 2

This smoothie is a treat for when you want something delectable. I eat it when I miss my grandmother Louise and her peach pies. If you want more protein, add half a block of raw silken tofu or 1/3 cup navy beans. You won't taste them.

- 1 cup plant milk (or 1/2 cup water and 1/2 cup plant milk)
- 1 banana
- 1 cup frozen or fresh peaches
- 1 Tablespoon ground flaxseeds
- 1 Tablespoon sweetener (stevia, maple syrup, etc)
- 1/4 teaspoon vanilla extract
- 1/4 teaspoon ground cinnamon
- pinch of ground ginger
- pinch of ground nutmeg

INSTRUCTIONS

1) Add all ingredients to a blender and blend on high for 45 seconds or until everything is equally smooth.

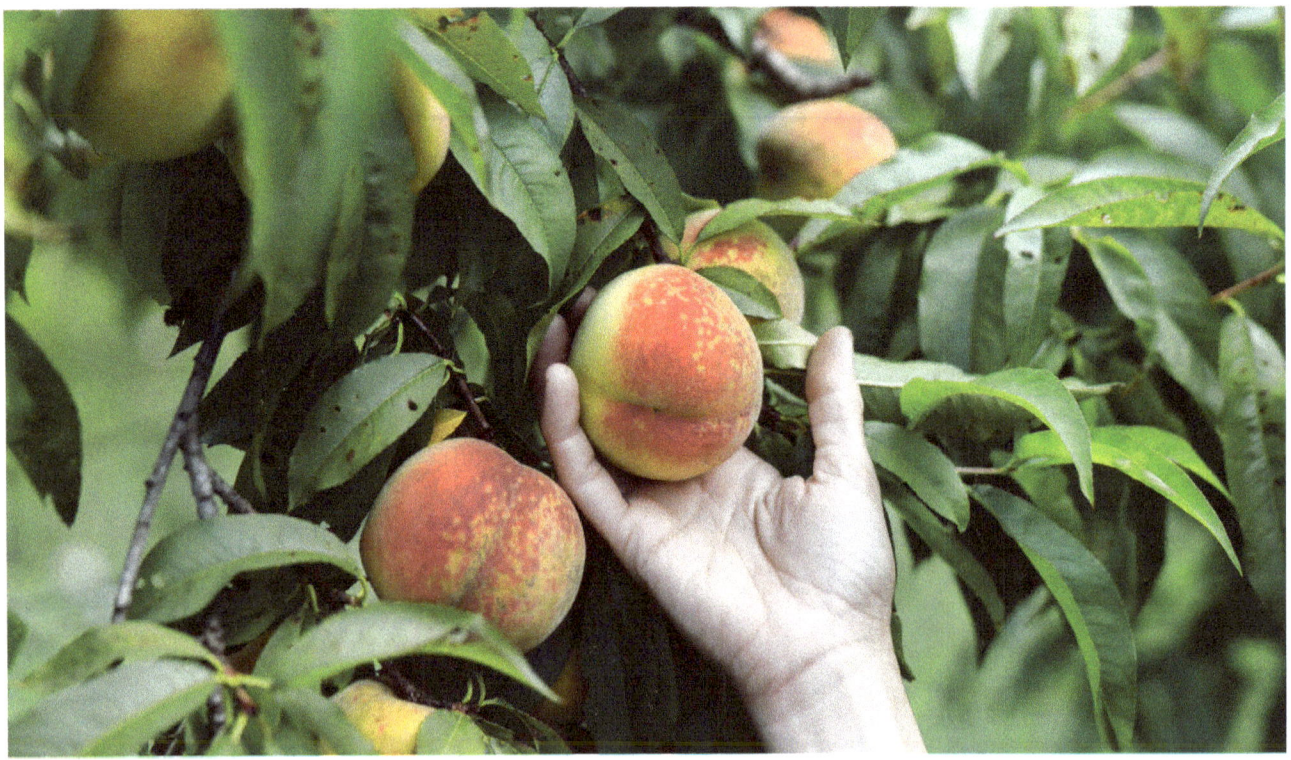

Chocolate Peanut Butter Smoothie

Servings: 2

This classic comforting smoothie flavor is an excellent way to get greens into children and/or to reward oneself for doing something hard. It is filled with greens, berries, nuts and seeds, yet tastes just like dessert. (If you use sweetened protein powder, try omitting the dates/ sweetener.)

- 1 banana, fresh or frozen
- 1/2 cup frozen leafy greens, or one large leaf of kale or collard greens, with the stem removed
- 1/2 cup blueberries, fresh or frozen
- 2 Tablespoons unsweetened cocoa powder
- 1 Tablespoon ground flaxseeds
- 2 big Tablespoons peanut butter
- 3 dates or 1 Tablespoon sweetener (maple syrup, sugar, etc)
- 1 cup water or ice
- 1 scoop chocolate protein powder, *optional*

INSTRUCTIONS

1) Add all ingredients to a blender and blend on high for 45 seconds or until everything is equally smooth.

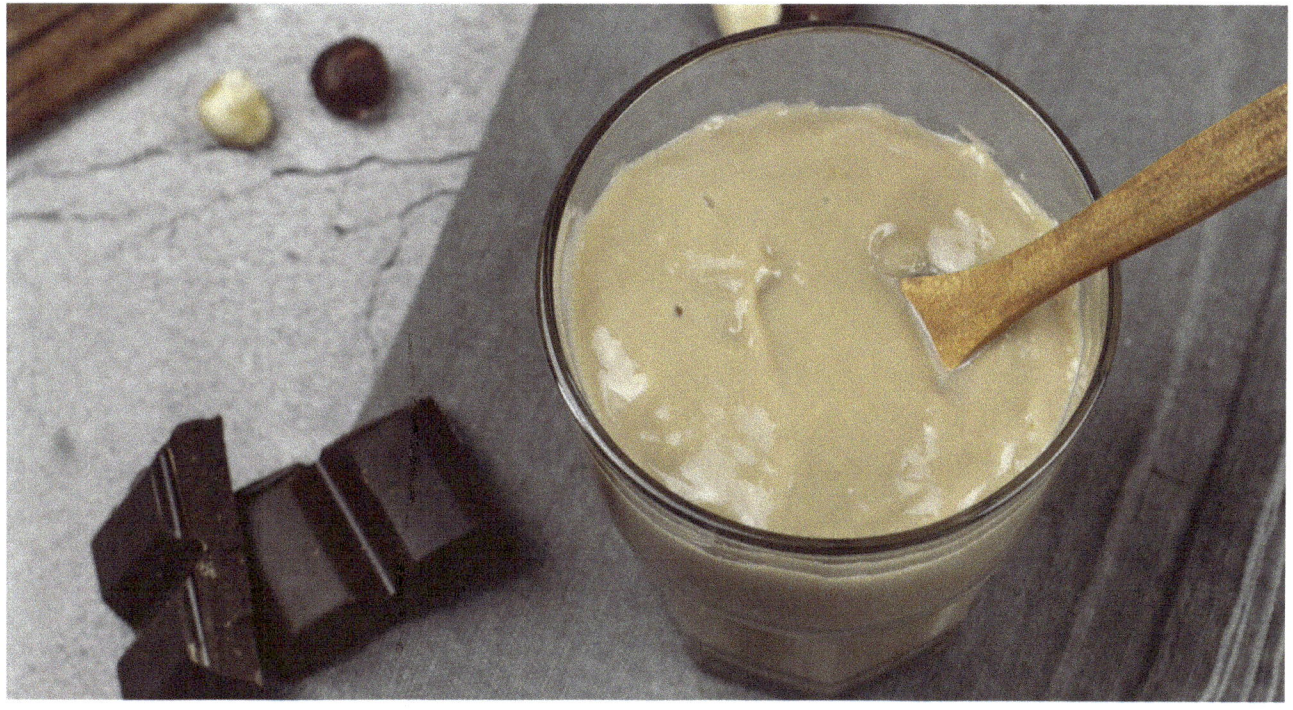

BREAKFAST

Magic Greens Smoothie

Servings: 3

This smoothie is refreshing. It's sweet from the dates and slightly tangy from the pineapple. The nutritional profile is dazzling–greens, fruits, healthy fats, fiber, citrus and spice all contributing benefits. Use a big blender jar rather than a bullet blender, which is a bit too small for this capacious recipe.

- 2 cups fresh baby spinach or 1 cup chopped frozen spinach
- 1 cup diced frozen pineapple
- 2/3 cup water or ice
- 1/2 of a banana
- 1/2 of an avocado
- 3 dates, pitted (or 1 Tablespoon sweetener)
- 1 Tablespoon ground flax seeds
- 1 teaspoon lemon juice
- 1/4 teaspoon ground ginger
- 1 scoop vanilla protein powder, *optional*

INSTRUCTIONS

1) Add all ingredients to a blender and blend on high for 45 seconds or until everything is equally smooth.

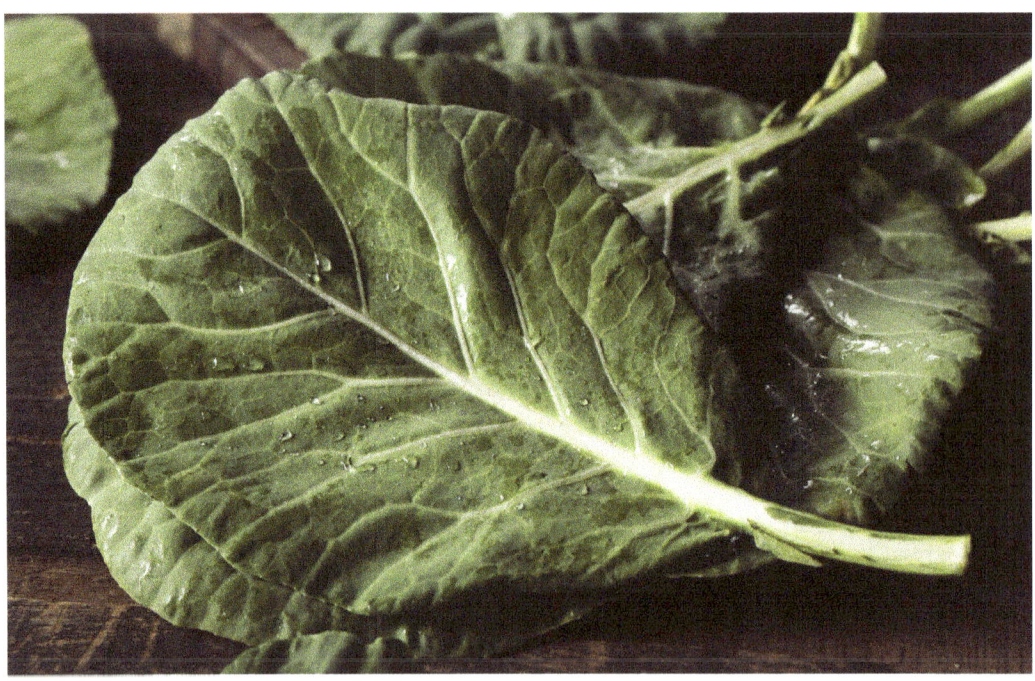

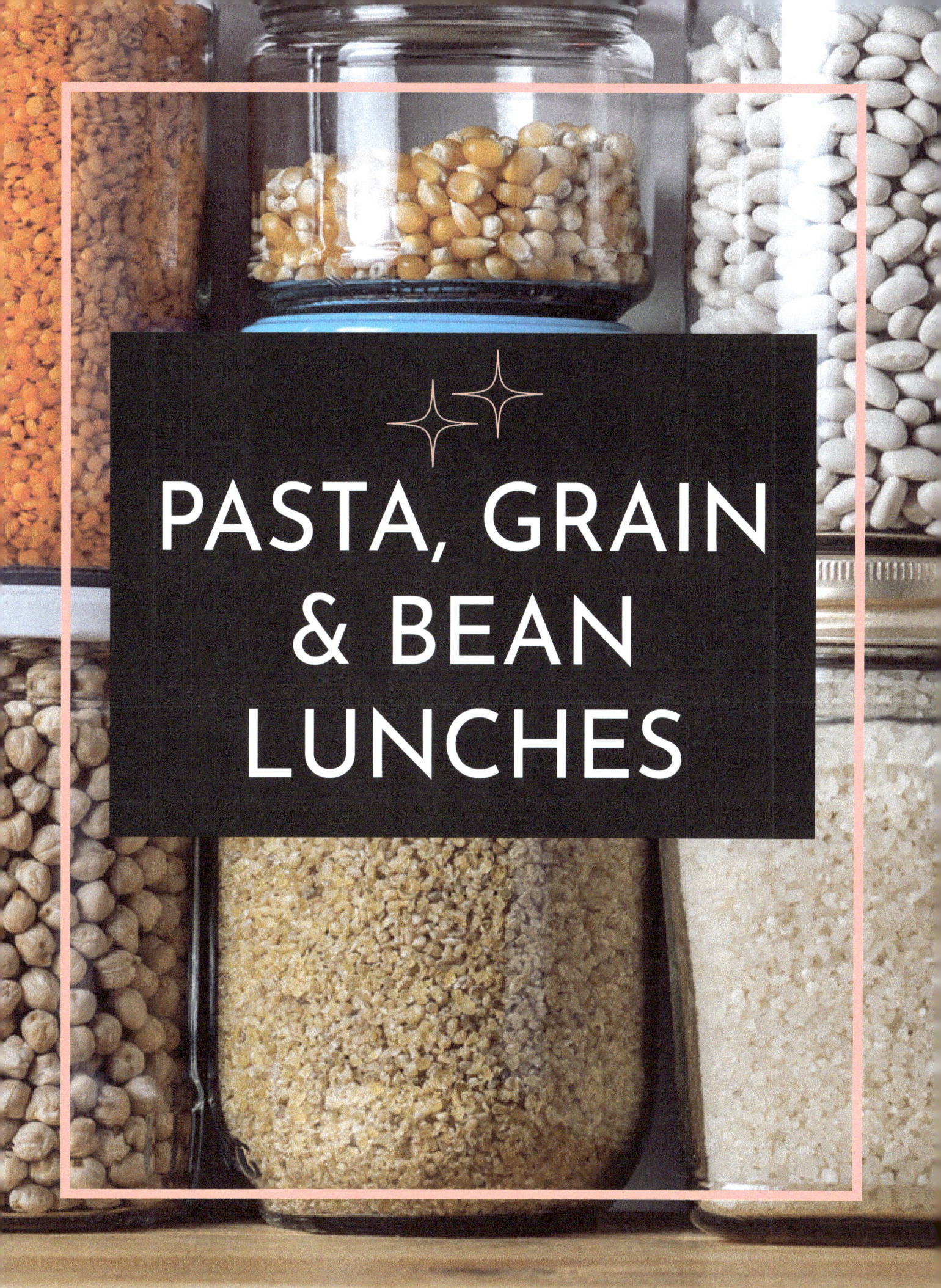

Pasta, Grain & Bean Lunches

Pasta with Red Lentil Tomato Sauce

Servings: 4

This dish is rich in protein, herbs and spices and flavor. If you need a fast and simple version, just add cooked red lentils and some herbs to an organic jarred tomato sauce spooned over your favorite pasta.

- 1 cup dried red lentils
- 3 cups water
- 1 28-oz jar of diced tomatoes, undrained, or 3-4 tomatoes diced
- 1 large red onion, chopped
- 4 garlic cloves, minced (or 1 Tablespoon dried minced garlic)
- 1/2 cup tomato paste or pizza sauce
- 2 Tablespoons olive oil, *optional*
- 1 Tablespoon white miso paste (or 1 Tablespoon soy sauce/tamari)
- 2 Tablespoons nutritional yeast
- 1 Tablespoon dried parsley
- 1.5 teaspoons dried basil
- 1 teaspoon dried oregano
- 1/2 teaspoon red pepper flakes
- 1 teaspoon sugar or 1 Tablespoon maple syrup
- 8-12 ounces whole grain or bean-based spaghetti

INSTRUCTIONS

1) Boil 2 cups water in a medium saucepot and add 1 cup red lentils. Turn heat down and simmer for 15-20 minutes or until lentils are soft and have lost their shape.

2) Chop onion and garlic. In a large pan over medium-low heat, sauté the onions and garlic in either 2 Tablespoons olive oil or the liquid from the can of tomatoes (if you avoid added oils). Cook for 5 minutes, adding more liquid if necessary. Then stir in the tomato paste/sauce, miso, nutritional yeast, basil, oregano, parsley, red pepper flakes and sugar/syrup.

3) Stir in 1 cup of water, then add the tomatoes and cooked lentils. Simmer the sauce, stirring frequently, for about 10 minutes, adding more water if desired. Taste and adjust seasonings as you like.

4) As the sauce is simmering, cook the spaghetti. Set a large pot of water on high heat to boil and add a pinch of salt. When water boils, add the spaghetti, stirring occasionally, for the amount of time specified on the bag. When it is al dente, drain spaghetti.

5) Serve the pasta with the sauce in equal amounts.

Pesto Garbanzo Pasta

Servings: 4-5

This brown rice pesto pasta sings with greens and garbanzo beans. It came together one day when I was looking in my pantry for something to cook and decided to improvise. Now, I make it at least once a month.

- 1 12 oz. bag Tinkyada brown rice pasta spirals
- 1 cup pesto (use vegan pesto recipe below or a jarred, store-bought pesto)
- 1.5 to 3 cups cooked garbanzo beans (chickpeas), or 1 to 2 cans rinsed and drained, as you prefer the ratio of beans to pasta
- 1/4 cup pumpkin seeds
- 1 to 2 Tablespoons sesame seeds
- 1/4 teaspoon red pepper flakes
- 1/2 to 1 teaspoon salt, to taste
- 1/2 teaspoon black pepper

Vegan Pesto Ingredients

- 2 cups fresh basil with large or woody stems removed (can substitute kale and add 1/2 tsp. sweetener, if you prefer)
- 3 Tablespoons pine nuts, walnuts, almonds or sunflower seeds
- 3 large cloves garlic, peeled
- 2 Tablespoons lemon juice
- 3-4 Tablespoons nutritional yeast (replaces Parmesan cheese flavor)
- 1/4 teaspoon sea salt, to taste
- 2-3 Tablespoons olive oil
- 3-5 Tablespoons water

INSTRUCTIONS

1) Soak 1 cup of dried garbanzo beans (chickpeas) overnight. Drain, rinse, and transfer to a pot. Cover with water twice the amount of beans and bring to a boil. Cover the pot, lower the heat and simmer for approximately one hour. Taste to make sure they're tender–if not, cook longer, up to another hour. Drain when they are done and allow to cool.

If you prefer the pressure cooker, add one part beans to two parts water and cook for 12 minutes on high with a 10-minute natural release.

2) Cook the brown rice pasta according to the instructions on the bag. My favorite way to cook it is the energy-saving method: add pasta to boiling water and cook for 2 minutes. Then remove from heat, cover, and let sit for 16-17 minutes. Drain pasta.

3) Pour the pasta back into the cooled pot. Add the pesto and stir well. Add the chickpeas, pumpkin seeds, sesame seeds, red pepper flakes, and salt/pepper to taste.

PESTO INSTRUCTIONS

1) Add the basil or kale, nuts, garlic, lemon juice, nutritional yeast, and salt to a blender or food processor and process on high for 45 seconds or until a loose paste comes together.

2) Add olive oil a little at a time. Scrape down sides as needed to ensure that everything mixes well. Then add 1 Tablespoon of water at a time until your desired consistency is reached – a thick but pourable sauce.

3) Taste pesto and adjust flavor to your preferences. Add more nutritional yeast for cheesy flavor, salt for overall flavor, nuts for nuttiness, garlic for bite/zing, or lemon juice for acidity.

4) Store leftovers covered in the refrigerator for up to 1 week or freeze the pesto for use over time.

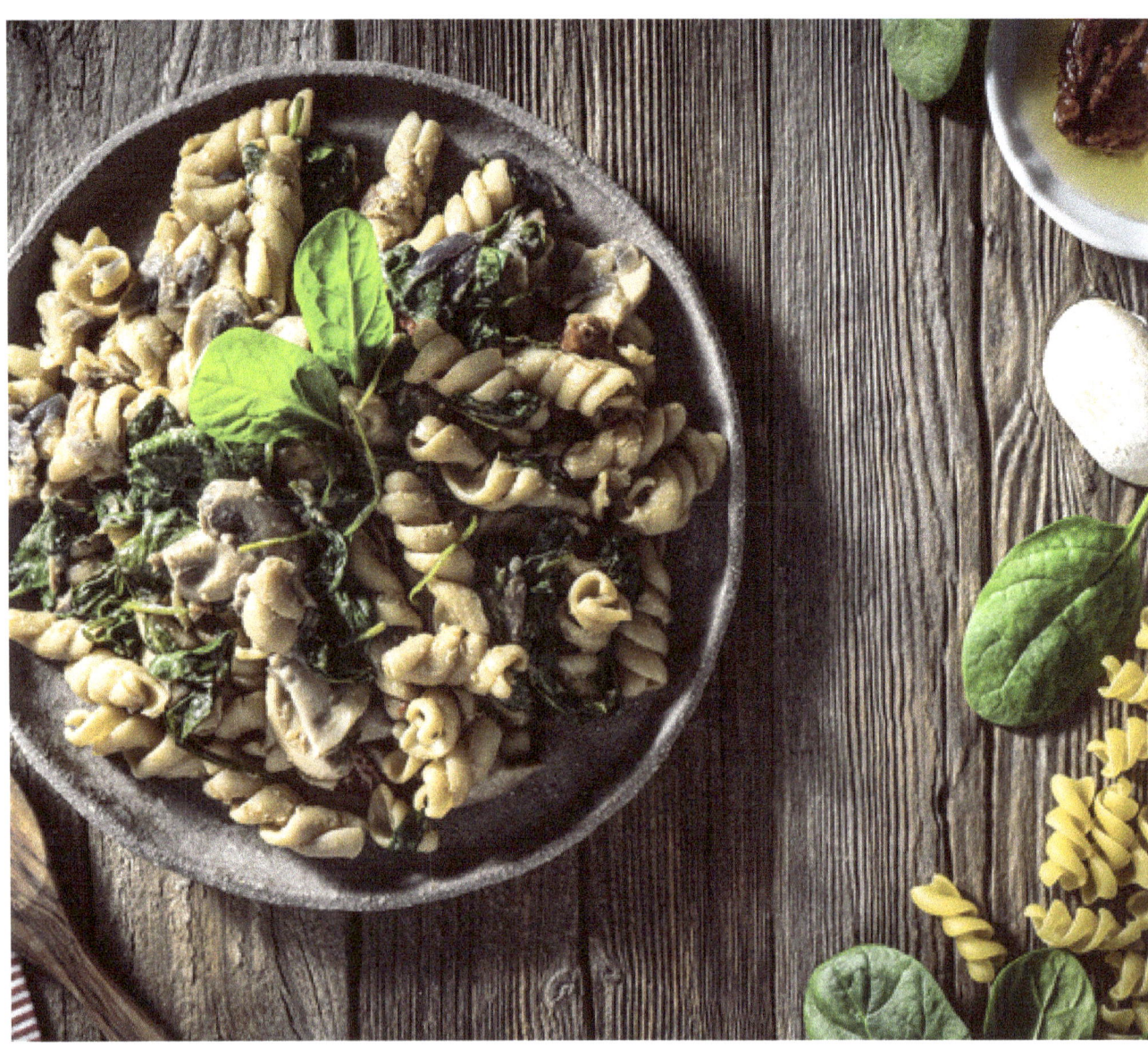

Peanut Saucy Noodles with White Beans and Scallions

Servings: 4

Noodles with peanut butter sauce are a scrumptious Asian staple! They're sweet and salty, fresh and energizing. If you have fresh ginger in the fridge, add a minced tablespoon to the recipe for even more kick.

- 12 oz of soba noodles, brown rice noodles, or whole wheat spaghetti
- 1.5 cups of cooked navy beans (or 1 can, drained and rinsed)
- 1 Tablespoon olive oil
- 1 Tablespoon sesame seeds
- 1/4 cup almond butter or peanut butter
- 1 carrot, grated
- 2 scallions, chopped
- 1 garlic clove, minced
- 2 teaspoons minced fresh ginger
- 1 Tablespoon lime juice
- 1 Tablespoon miso paste or soy sauce
- 1/2 teaspoon red pepper flakes
- 1/2 cup water

INSTRUCTIONS

1) Soak one cup of navy beans overnight, then drain, rinse and transfer to a cooking pot. To cook on the stovetop, cover with water three times the amount of beans and bring to a boil. Cover the pot, lower the heat and simmer for approximately one to two hours. Taste to make sure they're tender–if not, cook longer. Drain when they are done and allow to cool.

If you prefer the pressure cooker, add one part navy beans to two parts water and cook for 4 minutes on high with a 10-minute natural release. You will end up with 3 cups of cooked beans, though you only need 1.5 cups for this recipe. Save the rest in the freezer for adding to smoothies.

2) In a blender or food processor, add the almond/peanut butter, garlic, ginger, miso, lime juice and 1/2 cup water. Blend until smooth and creamy, adjusting water to reach the consistency you like best.

3) Cook the noodles according to the instructions, running them under cold water as soon as the cook time is complete. Drizzle them with olive oil and toss so they don't stick together.

4) Transfer the noodles to a large serving bowl and pour the nut butter dressing over the noodles. Add the shaved carrots and white beans and toss to mix everything well and coat all the noodles with the sauce. Sprinkle with scallions and sesame seeds and serve.

Sumptuous Alfredo Pasta with Summer Peas

Servings: 4

This vegan alfredo sauce is made of cashews and is a dairy-free alternative to alfredo sauce with a delicious, cheesy flavor. Soak the cashews the night before you want to make the recipe.

- 12 oz whole grain pasta
- 2 cups green peas
- 1 cup raw cashews, soaked overnight, drained and rinsed
- half of a yellow onion, diced fine
- 3/4 cup water
- 3 peeled garlic cloves
- 2 teaspoons lemon juice
- 2 Tablespoons nutritional yeast
- 1 teaspoon salt
- 1/4 to 1/2 teaspoon black pepper
- 1 Tablespoon black cumin (nigella sativa), ground, *optional*
- 1/2 to 1 cup pickled veggies, *optional*

INSTRUCTIONS

1) Soak the cashews overnight or for at least 6 hours, then drain and rinse them. If the green peas were frozen, defrost them by moving them from the freezer to the fridge the night before. If they're still too frosty when you're ready to cook, put them in a colander and run cool water over them for a minute or two.

2) Cook the pasta according to the package directions.

3) In a food processor or high-powered blender, combine the cashews, onion, water, garlic, lemon juice, nutritional yeast, salt and pepper. Process until smooth.

4) When the pasta is done, place the green peas in the bottom of the strainer and drain the pasta over it so the peas are warmed by the hot water and pasta. Transfer peas and pasta to a serving bowl, pour the alfredo sauce on top, and mix well to combine.

5) If you want this dish to be more complex, grind black cumin (nigella sativa) on top or add some quick-pickled veggies (see p. 87 for recipe).

New Orleans Style Red Beans and Rice

Servings: 4-6

This is my mother's recipe and I make it for guests more than any other dish. I use brown rice rather than the classic long-grain white rice, for the myriad nutrition benefits. If you use canned beans, the secret is to use Blue Runner Creole Cream Style Red Beans. I order them by the case to keep in the pantry.

- 5 cups cooked red beans (or 3 cans red beans drained and rinsed)
- 2 cups rinsed brown rice
- 5 cups water
- 1/2 large yellow onion, chopped fine
- 2 ribs celery, chopped fine
- 1/2 green pepper, chopped fine
- 6 cloves garlic, minced
- 2 Tablespoons olive oil
- 1 Tablespoon parsley
- 1 teaspoon salt
- 1 teaspoon basil
- 1 teaspoon oregano
- 1 teaspoon vegan Worcestershire sauce, *optional*
- 1/4 teaspoon cayenne pepper or 15 drops Tabasco sauce

INSTRUCTIONS

1) Pressure cook or stove cook 2 cups of dried red beans (or use 3 cans rinsed and drained red kidney beans, to end up with about 5 cups of cooked beans). To cook on the stove, add 2 cups red beans to 8 cups water, bring to a boil, then simmer for 2 hours. To pressure cook, add 2 cups red beans to 4 cups water. Set it for 7 minutes at high pressure with a ten-minute natural release. Taste for tenderness and add more time if needed.

2) To make brown rice, boil 4 cups water, add a splash of olive oil and pinch of salt. Add 2 cups rinsed brown rice. Simmer, covered, for 45 minutes, checking at 40 minutes for tenderness.

3) In a large pan, add 2 Tablespoons olive oil, chopped onion, bell pepper, celery, and garlic. Sauté for 5 minutes until soft.

4) Add your cooked beans and 1 cup water to the pan. Mash about half of the beans against the side of the pan with the back of a large spoon or use an immersion blender. Add the parsley, salt, basil, Worcestershire, Tabasco, or cayenne pepper.

5) Lower heat and cook, stirring frequently, for 10 minutes, adding water if needed.

6) Serve over brown rice.

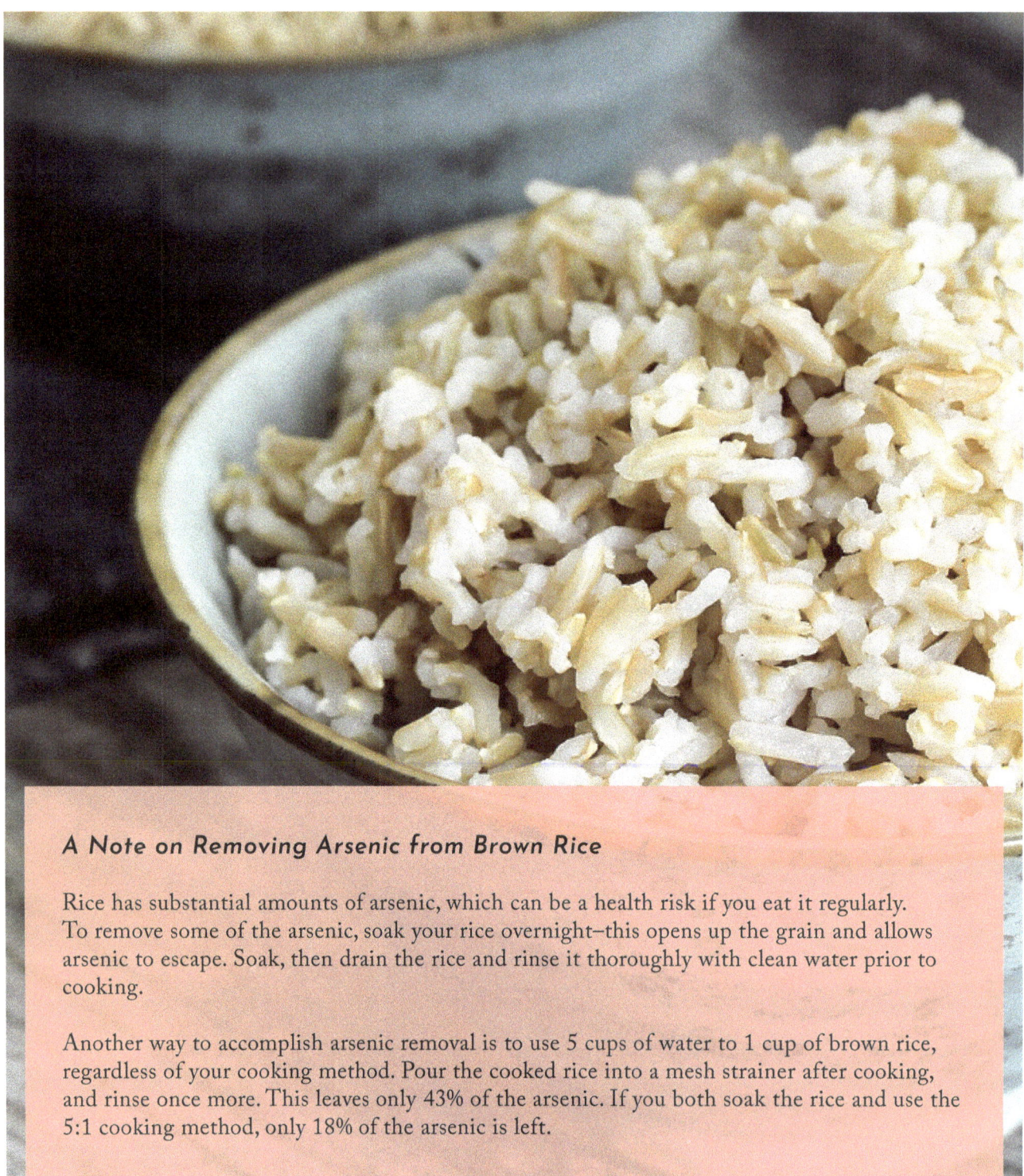

A Note on Removing Arsenic from Brown Rice

Rice has substantial amounts of arsenic, which can be a health risk if you eat it regularly. To remove some of the arsenic, soak your rice overnight—this opens up the grain and allows arsenic to escape. Soak, then drain the rice and rinse it thoroughly with clean water prior to cooking.

Another way to accomplish arsenic removal is to use 5 cups of water to 1 cup of brown rice, regardless of your cooking method. Pour the cooked rice into a mesh strainer after cooking, and rinse once more. This leaves only 43% of the arsenic. If you both soak the rice and use the 5:1 cooking method, only 18% of the arsenic is left.

Spicy Bean Macaroni Salad

Servings: 7

This tangy salad is reminiscent of summer picnics and packs a lot of protein, fiber, iron and essential minerals into your lunch. It uses canned beans so you can have a variety of beans with quick preparation time.

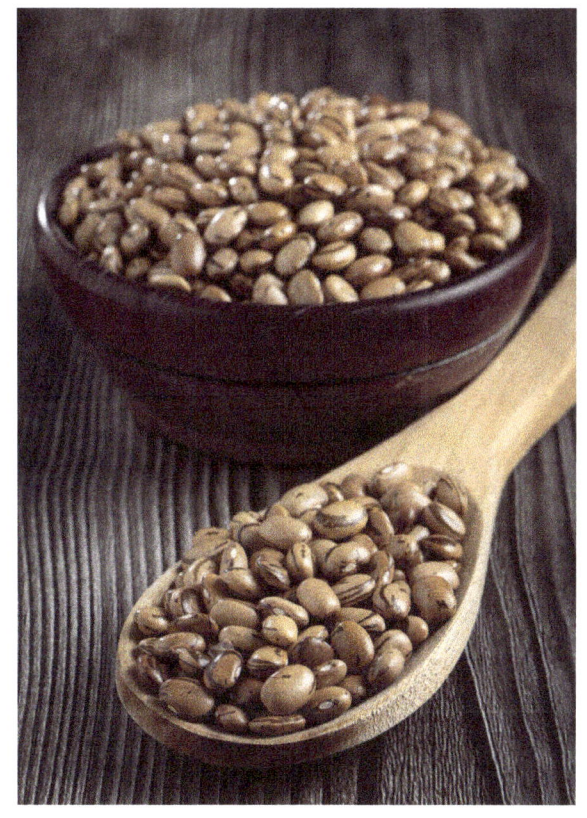

- 1 lb whole wheat or bean-based macaroni
- 1 can each of pinto beans, kidney beans, and chickpeas, rinsed and drained
- 1 medium red onion, diced
- 3 Tablespoons red wine vinegar
- 1 Tablespoon vegan mayonnaise
- 1 teaspoon or Tablespoon Dijon mustard, to taste
- 1 teaspoon red pepper flakes
- 1 teaspoon balsamic vinegar
- 1 teaspoon maple syrup

INSTRUCTIONS

1) In a large pot, cook macaroni according to package instructions. Drain and rinse.

2) Mix 3 cans of drained, rinsed beans into the pasta. (Or, if you have various cooked beans, mix 4 cups cooked beans into the pasta.)

2) Add 1 diced red onion, 1 Tablespoon vegan mayo, 3 Tablespoons red wine vinegar, 1 teaspoon or Tablespoon Dijon mustard to taste, 1 teaspoon red pepper flakes, 1 teaspoon balsamic vinegar and 1 teaspoon maple syrup. Stir well.

3) Before eating, throw in some baby greens or chopped romaine lettuce to your bowl and stir. Enjoy a crisp and refreshing bean pasta salad!

Cranberry Quinoa with Green Peas

Servings: 6

Quinoa is a high-protein seed cultivated by the ancient Incas. It works like a grain in meals. Be sure to rinse your quinoa in a mesh strainer until the water runs clear, or it will taste bitter. The saponins on the exterior of the quinoa, which protect it from insect predators, may give you a tummy ache. Rinsed cooked quinoa is sweet, light, and nutty. Quinoa quadruples in size when cooked.

- 1 cup quinoa, rinsed and drained
- 2 cups water or veggie stock
- 1 cup green peas (can also use canned or cooked black-eyed peas)
- 1/2 cup cranberries or raisins
- 1/2 cup slivered almonds
- 1 carrot, grated, *optional*

Easy Seasoning Option

If not using veggie stock, add the following to 2 cups water:

- 1 Tablespoon concentrated stock such as Better Than Bouillon vegetable or roasted garlic flavor
- 1 Tablespoon minced dehydrated garlic or 3 cloves minced fresh garlic
- 1 Tablespoon minced dehydrated chives or onion, or 1/2 onion chopped fine

Spice Variety Seasoning Option

If not using veggie stock or easy seasoning option, add the following to 2 cups water:

- 1 teaspoon brown sugar, maple syrup or stevia
- 2 teaspoons lemon juice
- 1 teaspoon cumin seeds or 1/2 teaspoon ground cumin
- 1 teaspoon smoked paprika
- 1 teaspoon white miso paste, *optional*
- 1/2 teaspoon nutritional yeast
- 1/4 teaspoon dried parsley
- 1/2 teaspoon garlic powder
- 1/4 teaspoon dried mustard
- 1/4 teaspoon ground turmeric
- 1/4 teaspoon dried basil
- 1/4 teaspoon onion powder

INSTRUCTIONS

1) Add quinoa to a mesh strainer and rinse thoroughly under running water for 2 minutes.

2) Add frozen green peas, cranberries, and almonds to two cups water/stock in a medium pot. Bring water/veggie stock to a boil. If using Easy Seasoning recipe, add all other ingredients to the pot.

3) Add one cup quinoa, cover, reduce heat and simmer for 20 minutes. At twenty minutes, remove from heat and uncover.

4) If using Spice Variety Seasoning option, in a large serving bowl, combine lemon juice, sugar/syrup/sweetener, all spices and white miso paste. Whisk together.

5) Pour cooked quinoa medley into large bowl with grated carrot and all other ingredients. Toss well to mingle flavors. Serve and enjoy.

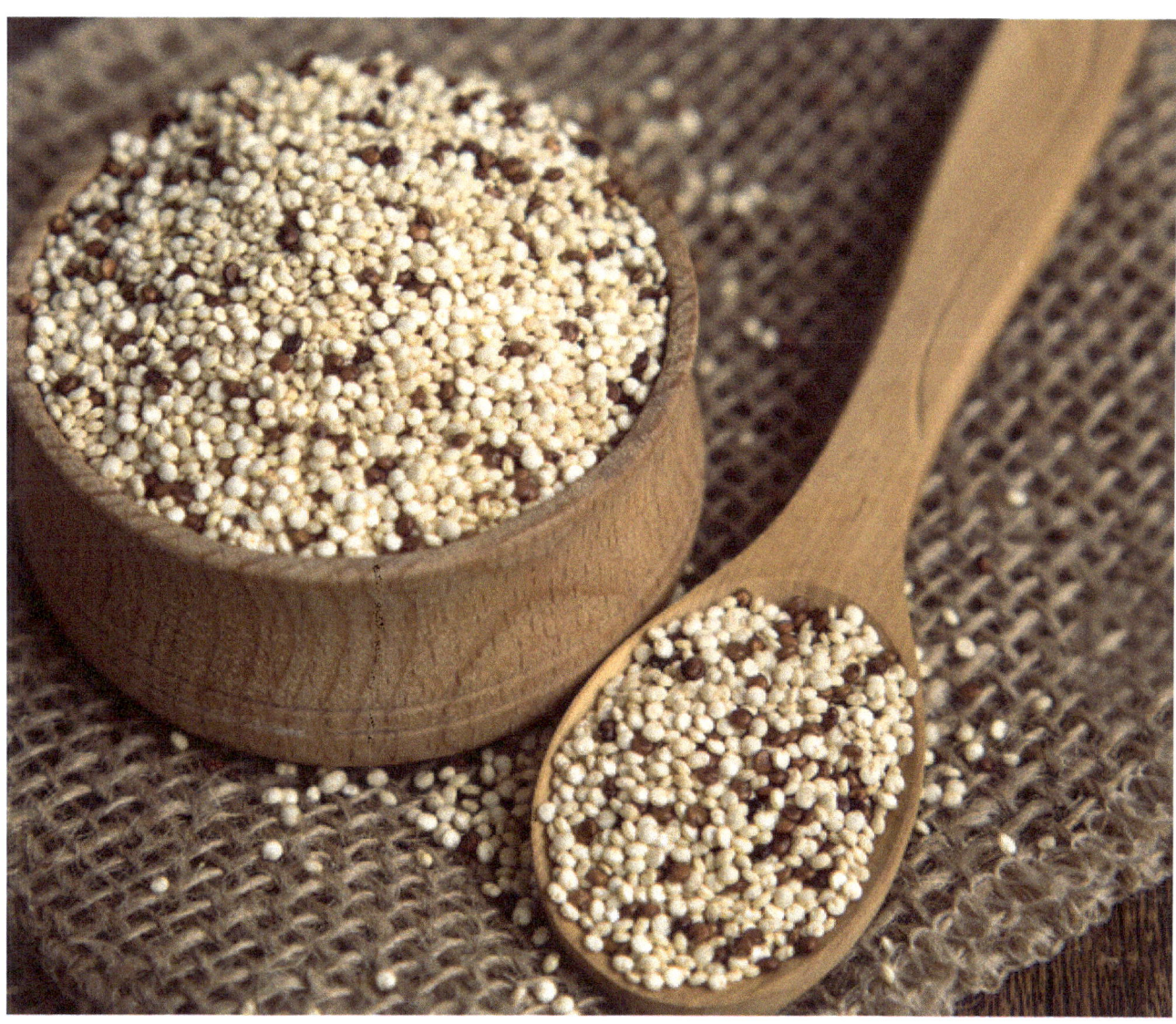

PASTA, GRAIN AND BEAN LUNCH DISHES

A Perfect Sandwich

When you need an impromptu lunch, a sandwich is the classic choice. Sturdy whole grain bread, thickly spread hummus, sweet or tart sliced apples and bright spears of red onion. The crisp, sweet and earthy combo is refreshing and full of contrast. Have it open-faced, or closed if you need it to travel.

    2 slices of whole grain bread

    hummus, about 4 Tablespoons

    one green or red apple

    one quarter of a red onion, sliced into thin spears

    freshly ground pepper and a pinch of salt to taste

INSTRUCTIONS

1) Slice the apple into quarters around the core and discard the core. Slice each quarter into thinner slices. Slice the quarter of a red onion into thin spears.

2) Spread hummus on each slice of bread, toasted if you prefer. On top of the hummus, layer the apple slices and red onion spears. Salt and pepper if you like.

Optional: add fresh sprouts

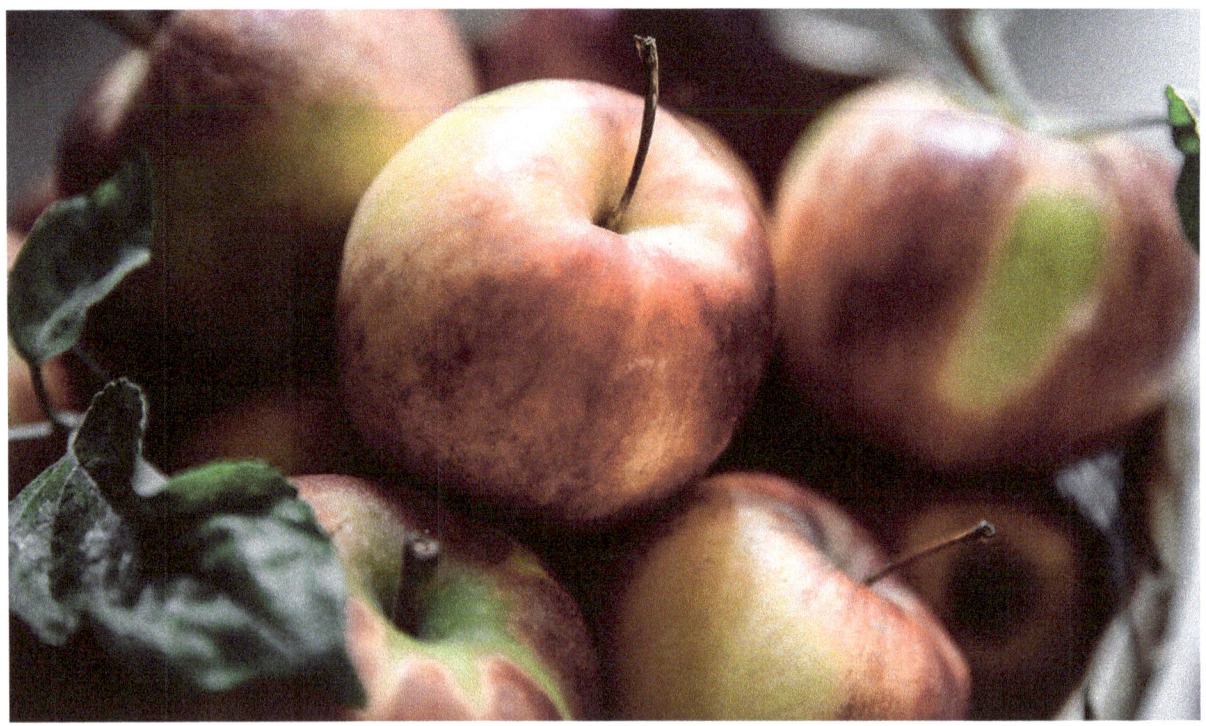

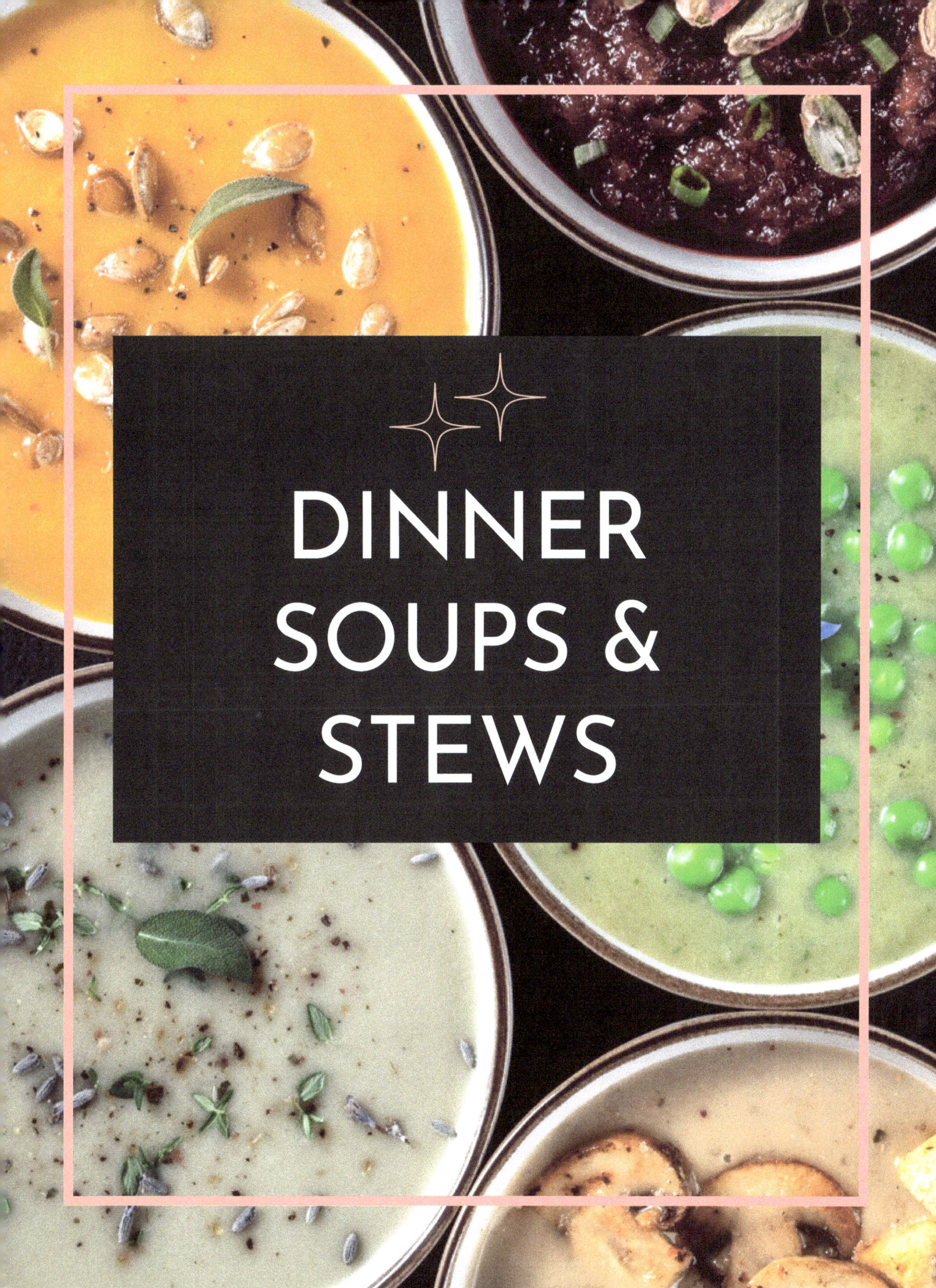

DINNER SOUPS & STEWS

Spicy Red Lentil Soup

Servings: 4

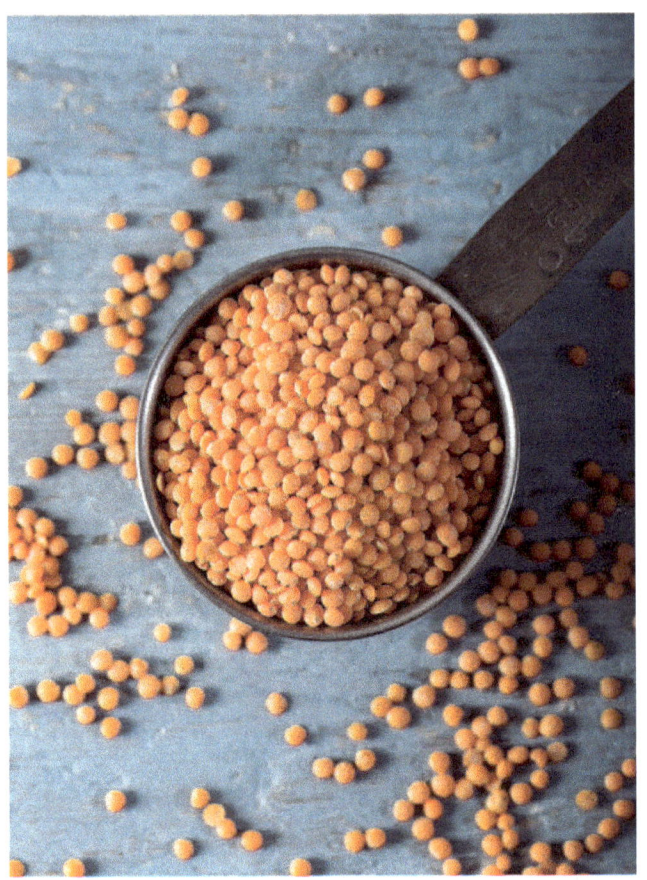

1.5 cups red lentils
5 cups water or vegetable broth
3 cloves of garlic, minced or pressed
1 medium red or yellow onion, chopped
1.5 heaping Tablespoons curry powder
1.5 teaspoons ginger, fresh or powdered
1/4 teaspoon cayenne pepper
1 bay leaf
1 teaspoon lemon juice
1/2-1 teaspoon salt, to taste

INSTRUCTIONS

1) In a pot on the stovetop, bring water/broth to a boil. Add red lentils, onion, garlic, curry powder, ginger, cayenne pepper, bay leaf, lemon juice. Lower heat and cook for 20-30 minutes or until the lentils drop their outlines and become soft.

2) In the last five minutes of cooking, you can add any extra veggies you like and have on hand such as chopped kale or tomatoes. Add salt to taste.

3) Serve in a bowl, and garnish with pumpkin seeds, vegan sour cream, or chopped peanuts.

Green Curry Tofu and Vegetables

Servings: 4-5

This is a simple version of a Thai green curry dish and takes about 30 minutes, using jarred green curry paste and coconut milk, available at the grocery store. If you made brown rice ahead of time, warm it to serve with the curry. Otherwise, cook 1.5 cups of rinsed brown rice in 3 cups of water in a separate pot while you make this mouth-watering curry.

- 4 to 6 Tablespoons jarred green curry paste
- 1 Tablespoon oil, *optional*
- 1 medium yellow onion, chopped fine
- 6 ounces mushrooms, sliced
- 5 large cloves garlic, minced
- 1 small finger-size piece ginger root, peeled and minced or zested, or 1 Tablespoon ground ginger
- 1 package extra-firm tofu, patted or pressed dry, cut into small cubes
- 1 large red bell pepper, thinly sliced or diced
- 1 broccoli or cauliflower crown, cut into small florets
- 2 handfuls fresh snow peas, *optional*
- 1 can regular coconut milk
- 1/2 can lite coconut milk or water
- 1 Tablespoon arrowroot starch or corn starch
- 1 teaspoon fine sea salt
- 1 teaspoon lime juice

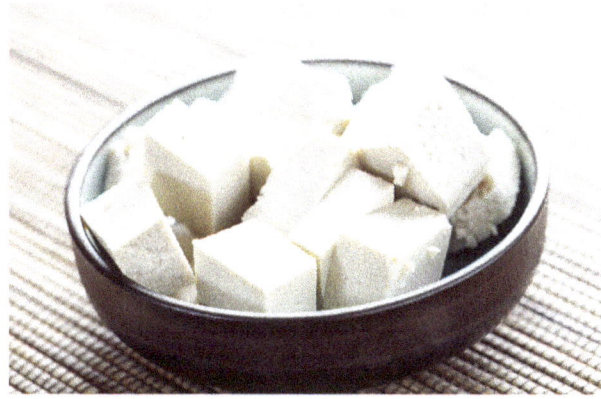

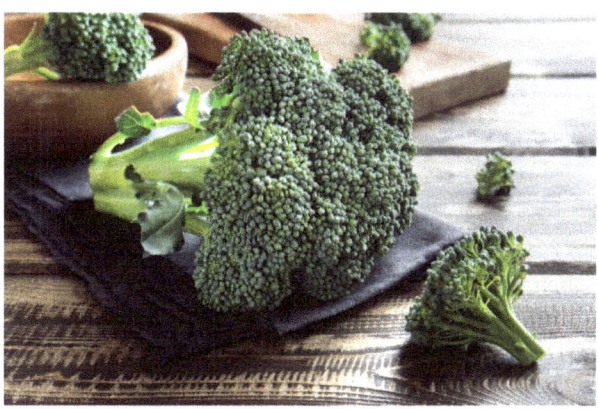

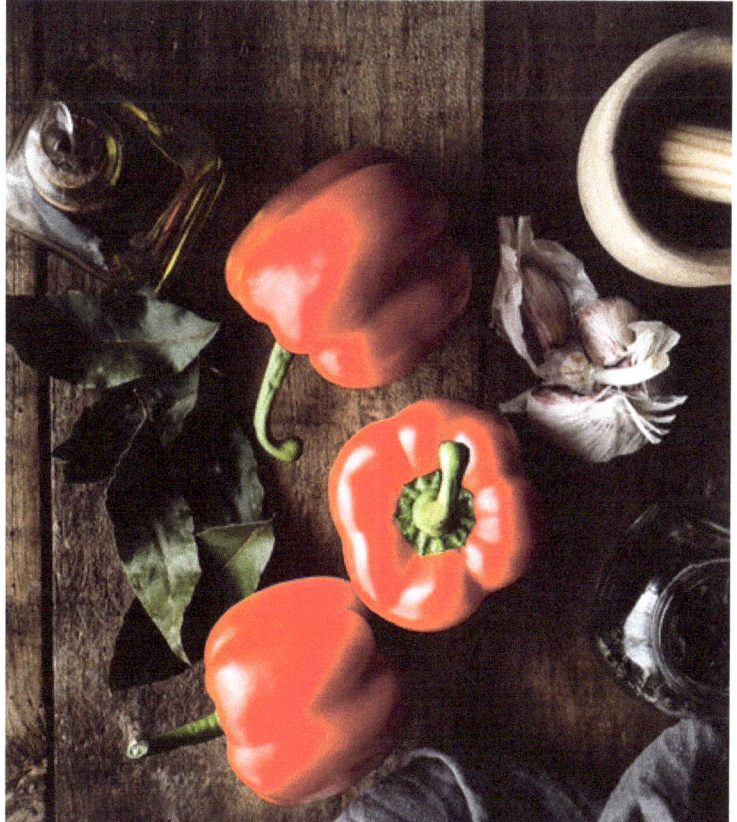

INSTRUCTIONS

1) Chop your veggies before you start cooking, so that you can put everything in the pan in order.

2) Heat a large skillet over medium-low heat. Add oil and green curry paste. If not using oil, add green curry paste and 1 Tablespoon of water. Stir and cook for about a minute.

3) Turn the heat up to medium and add the onion and mushrooms. Cook about 3 minutes.

4) Add the ginger, garlic, and tofu. Cook for about 5 minutes, stirring occasionally. Add more water or oil as needed to keep ingredients from sticking to the pan.

5) Add the broccoli or cauliflower, red bell pepper, and snow peas. Cook for 2 more minutes. Add the lime juice.

6) Add the can of regular coconut milk to the pan. Then take half of the can of lite coconut milk (or half a cup of water) and dissolve the arrowroot powder or corn starch in the can or cup. Add this slurry to the pan and turn up the heat to bring the dish to a low boil.

7) Reduce the heat to a simmer. Cook for about 4 minutes more or until the sauce has thickened and the vegetables are at just right tenderness.

8) Serve with brown rice.

African Peanut Yam Soup

Servings: 6

This is the most involved soup in this guide, and it will reward you. If you have them around, you can use already-baked sweet potatoes and cut down on cooking time. This is a spicy, fragrant, potent, creamy, intense, nourishing soup rich in antioxidants, protein and fiber.

- 4 cups veggie broth (or water with bouillon)
- 1 onion, chopped
- 1 or 2 yams or sweet potatoes, peeled and chopped into small cubes
- 2 Tablespoons fresh minced ginger or 1 Tablespoon powdered ginger
- 2 or 3 carrots, chopped into cubes
- 1.5 cups cooked chickpeas (1 can drained and rinsed, or equivalent pressure cooked)
- 1.5 cups of tomatoes, diced
- 1 cup peanut butter (unsweetened, if possible)
- 2 diced, deseeded jalapeños
- 5 garlic cloves, pressed or minced
- 1/4 to 1/2 teaspoon cayenne pepper, to taste
- 1/2 teaspoon black pepper
- 1 teaspoon ground coriander
- 1 teaspoon salt to taste
- 1 pinch cloves
- splash of lime juice to taste, *optional*
- some chopped peanuts for topping

INSTRUCTIONS

1) If cooking beans, soak one cup of chickpeas (garbanzo beans) overnight, then drain, rinse and transfer to a pot. On the stovetop, cover with water 3 times the amount of beans, bring to a boil, cover, lower the heat and simmer for 60 to 90 minutes. Taste to make sure they're tender–if not, cook longer. If using the pressure cooker, add one part chickpeas to two parts water and cook for 15 minutes on high with a 10-minute natural release.

2) In a big soup pot, heat a Tablespoon of olive oil or 1/3 cup broth or water and add onions. Sauté onions over medium heat for 10 minutes, adding more water as necessary to keep the onions from sticking. Add the garlic. Chop the sweet potatoes and carrots and add, stirring. Add more broth or water to keep veggies from sticking. Mix in all other ingredients except the 3 cups water/broth and the peanut butter: add the jalapeños, tomatoes, and spices. Continue to cook, stirring frequently, for 5 minutes.

3) Add the water/broth. Bring to a boil, reduce heat and simmer for 20-30 minutes or until the sweet potatoes are soft. Turn off heat. Add the peanut butter.

4) Blend soup well with an immersion blender or pour it into a regular blender in several portions and blend till smooth. Taste and adjust spices. If you like, you could add a little coconut milk or soy milk. If you like a thinner soup, add a little more broth.

5) Serve in a bowl and top with chopped peanuts.

Barley-Mushroom Soup with Tofu

Servings: 6

A Jewish classic, this hearty soup is updated with tofu to add more protein and a great dose of isoflavones. The pearl barley is a hearty grain that will keep you going for hours, and the mushrooms impart a savory umami sensation.

- 1 cup pearled barley
- 1/2 to 1 block firm tofu, chopped into 1/2-inch cubes
- 1 yellow onion, chopped
- 2 carrots, diced
- 1 pound mushrooms, sliced
- 1/2 cup dried shiitake mushrooms, soaked, *optional*
- 4 cloves garlic, diced
- 5-6 cups veggie stock, preferably low sodium
- 3 Tablespoons soy sauce/tamari
- 1 Tablespoon dried parsley
- 3/4 teaspoon thyme
- 1/2 teaspoon black pepper
- splash of sherry or vermouth, *optional*

INSTRUCTIONS

1) Chop the onions and carrots and mince the garlic. In a large soup pot, add a little olive oil or broth and sauté the onions and carrots for 5 minutes. Add the garlic and mushrooms, stirring frequently, and sauté for another 5 minutes.

2) Add the veggie stock, 1 Tablespoon dried parsley, 3 Tablespoon soy sauce, black pepper, thyme, and splash of sherry or vermouth. Taste for level of salt. If not fully salty already, add 1/2 to 1 teaspoon salt. Bring to a simmer.

3) Add 1 cup pearled barley and 1/2 to 1 full block of tofu, depending on how you like the tofu ratio. Stir. Bring back to a simmer, then turn to low and cook for 40-50 minutes. Serve when hot and store the rest in a 64-oz Mason jar.

Broccoli Cheeze Soup

Servings: 5

This soup is a comforting classic, in the vegan version. The broccoli gives a wonderful dose of protein and cancer-preventing compounds while the nutritional yeast imparts the cheesy flavor and delivers your daily dose of many B vitamins. I like to have this soup in a mug, by a rainy window, with a book, a cat and a blanket.

- 4–5 large carrots, chopped
- 1 cup veggie broth or water
- 1 large potato, peeled and chopped
- 3 cups broccoli florets,
- 3 cups vegetable broth
- 1/2 onion, chopped
- 2 stalks celery, chopped
- 1/4 cup nutritional yeast
- 2 cloves garlic, minced
- 2 cups soymilk or nut milk
- 1.5 teaspoons salt, to taste
- 2 Tablespoons olive oil

INSTRUCTIONS

1) In a large pan, heat olive oil or 1/2 cup water or broth, then add the onion, celery, carrots and potatoes. Sauté for 5 minutes, add the garlic and sauté for 5 minutes more. Add more water as needed to keep the vegetables from sticking to the pan.

2) Add the vegetable broth, broccoli and plant-based milk. Simmer for 5 minutes or until broccoli is vivid green.

3) Using an immersion blender or a high-speed blender, blend the soup until it is creamy. Add more liquid if it is too thick for you, 1/2 cup at a time.

4) Add nutritional yeast and salt and stir well. Serve with whole grain bread and green salad. Store the rest in a 64-oz Mason jar.

Yellow Split Pea Soup (Matar Dal)

Servings: 6

This traditional Indian soup is highly medicinal due to the intense spices, and is nourishing and comforting. This recipe is my attempt to replicate the soup at my favorite neighborhood Indian restaurant, where it is served in tiny steel bowls before meals.

- 6 cups water or veggie broth
- 2 cups yellow split peas, soaked 4 hours or overnight
- 1 onion, chopped (or 1/2 cup dehydrated)
- 3-5 cloves garlic (or 1 Tablespoon dehydrated)
- 1 Tablespoon ginger
- 1 Tablespoon turmeric, *optional*
- 1 teaspoon cumin
- 1 teaspoon coriander
- 1 teaspoon salt, to taste
- 1/2 teaspoon cayenne
- 1/2 teaspoon basil
- 1/2 teaspoon parsley
- juice of 1 lemon

Optional Veggies to Add:
- *kale*
- *carrots*
- *potatoes*
- *sweet potatoes*

INSTRUCTIONS

1) Soak the yellow split peas for 4 hours or overnight.

2) Sauté onion and any other veggies you like in olive oil, or 1/4 to 1/2 cup water or broth for 5-10 minutes.

3) Add all ingredients to the pressure cooker. Set for 15 minutes at high pressure. Do a natural release for 10 minutes. Or, if you prefer to cook on the stovetop, simmer for 40-50 minutes until tender. *Optional: puree with immersion blender to make it smoother.*

4) Serve with a dollop of vegan sour cream or cashew cream.

Black Bean, Kale & Butternut Squash Stew in the Slow Cooker

Servings: 6

This soup benefits from being cooked in a slow cooker to marry all the flavors. The InstantPot has both a sauté function and a slow cooker function, so you can use that appliance for everything, or use a separate sauté pan and slow cooker. You can also cook this dish in a regular soup pot on the stove, simmering for 30 minutes, or in the Instant Pot on high pressure for 17 minutes with a natural release.

- 1 lb butternut squash, peeled and cut into 1/2-inch cubes
- 3 cups cooked black beans (or two cans, drained and rinsed)
- 3.5 cups water or veggie stock
- 1.5 cups diced tomatoes
- 1 bunch kale or other greens, washed and chopped to ribbons or small pieces
- 1 yellow onion, chopped
- 1 red bell pepper, chopped
- 2 garlic cloves
- 1 fresh hot chile or jalapeño, minced
- 1 Tablespoon maple syrup
- 1 teaspoon allspice
- 2 bay leaves
- 1 teaspoon salt

INSTRUCTIONS

1) To cook black beans on the stove, soak for 4 hours or overnight, then simmer 1 cup beans in 3 cups water or vegetable broth for 1.5 hours. To cook black beans in a pressure cooker, add one cup beans and 1.75 cups water to the cooker. Set it for 6 to 8 minutes at high pressure, with a 10-minute natural release. Taste to make sure they're tender, and if not, cook for a little more time.

2) Sauté the onion, bell pepper, garlic in a skillet for five minutes in 1/3 cup extra water or broth, or a little oil.

3) Add cooked veggies to the slow cooker. Add the butternut squash, black beans, broth, spices and all other ingredients except your kale greens. Cook on low for 4 to 6 hours or on high for 2 to 3 hours, to taste.

4) In the last 5 minutes, add your chopped greens and stir to combine.

Classic Black Bean Soup

Servings: 5

This Latin-inspired soup is simple and hearty. Once you have it in your bowl, you can melt some vegan mozzarella on top with a few minutes under the toaster oven broiler to make it even more scrumptious. If you like cilantro, add some fresh chopped cilantro on top.

- 1 medium yellow or red onion, diced
- 2 medium carrots, diced
- 1 green bell pepper, de-seeded and diced
- 1 tomato, diced
- 2 ribs celery, diced
- 3 cloves garlic, minced
- 2 Tablespoons olive oil
- 2 teaspoons cumin
- 1 teaspoon dried oregano
- 2 teaspoons chili powder
- 1/2 teaspoon coriander powder
- 1/4 teaspoon cayenne pepper
- 3–4 cups vegetable broth
- 1 cup tomato sauce (any tomato pasta sauce works)
- 3 cups cooked black beans (or 2 cans, drained and rinsed)
- 1 Tablespoon maple syrup
- salt and pepper, to taste
- squeeze of fresh lime juice

INSTRUCTIONS

1) If cooking beans, soak 1.5 cups of black beans in 6 cups water overnight. Rinse, drain and transfer to a pot. On the stovetop, cover beans with 2 inches of water and bring to a boil. Lower heat, cover and simmer until tender, or 1.5 to 2 hours, adding more water if needed. If using a pressure cooker, add beans and 4 cups water and cook for 10 minutes on high pressure with a natural release.

2) Add the onion, carrot, bell pepper, celery, and garlic to a large soup pot with 2 Tablespoons of olive oil (use vegetable broth if avoiding oil). Sauté over medium heat for 5-7 minutes until fragrant and softened.

3) Stir in the tomato, cumin, oregano, coriander, cayenne pepper and chili powder and cook for 2-3 more minutes.

4) Add the vegetable broth, tomato sauce and black beans and bring the soup to a light simmer. Simmer lightly, uncovered, about 15 minutes.

5) In two portions, pour soup into a blender or food processor and blend until smooth. Be careful to allow steam to escape when blending. You can also use an immersion blender. If you prefer soup to be chunkier, only blend half. If you like it smooth, blend away.

6) Stir in the lime juice. Taste and adjust seasonings and salt and pepper, if needed.

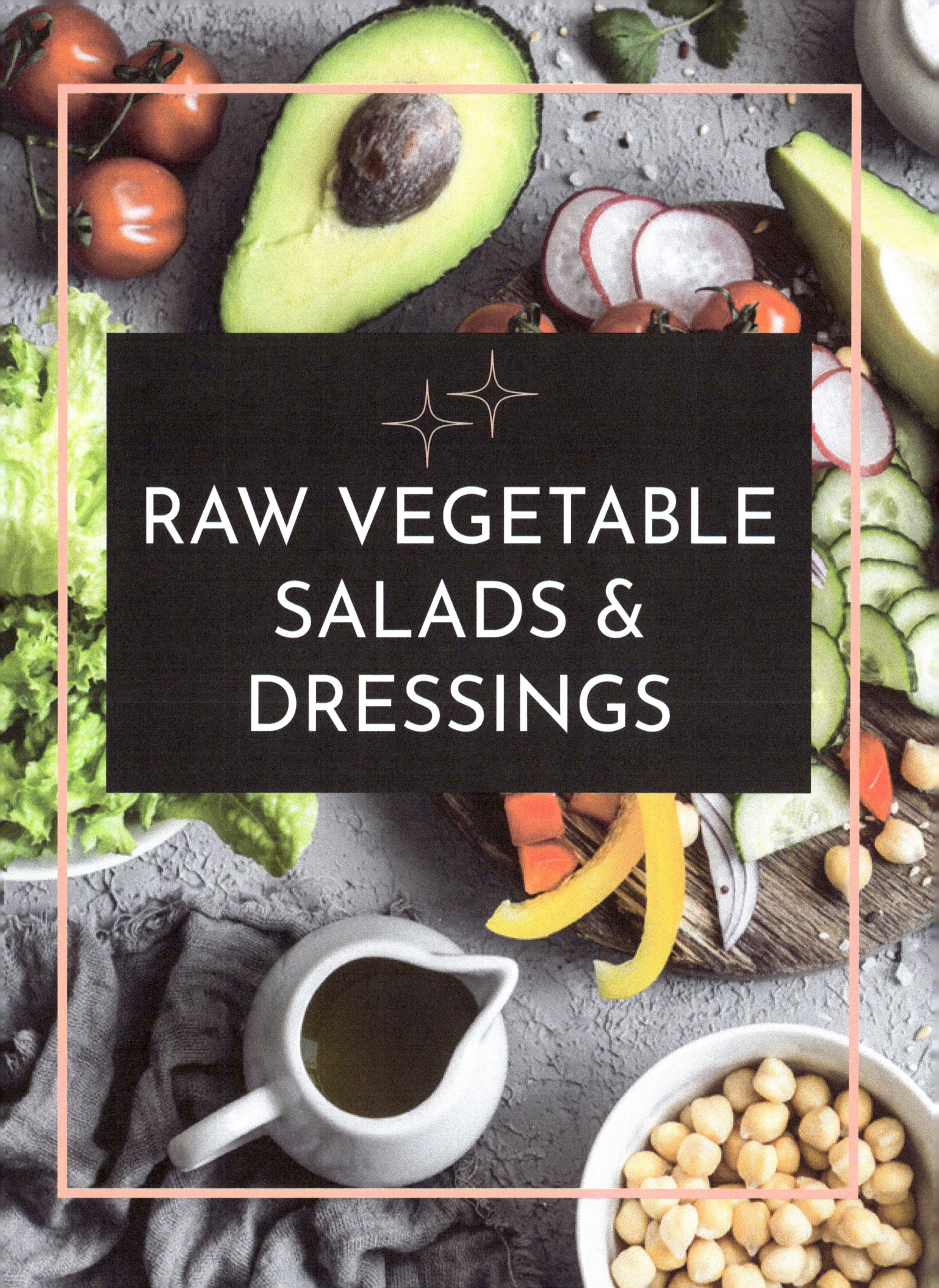

RAW VEGETABLE SALADS & DRESSINGS

Coleslaw with Miso Ginger Tamari Dressing

For the Coleslaw

1/2 head of green or red cabbage, chopped up

3 carrots diced

1 Tablespoon sesame seeds or chia seeds

For the Miso Ginger Tamari Dressing

2 Tablespoons rice vinegar

2 Tablespoons tahini (sesame butter)

2 teaspoons lemon juice

2 teaspoons maple syrup

1 teaspoon ginger (fresh or powdered)

1 teaspoon white miso paste or
   1 teaspoon tamari/soy sauce

2 teaspoons water

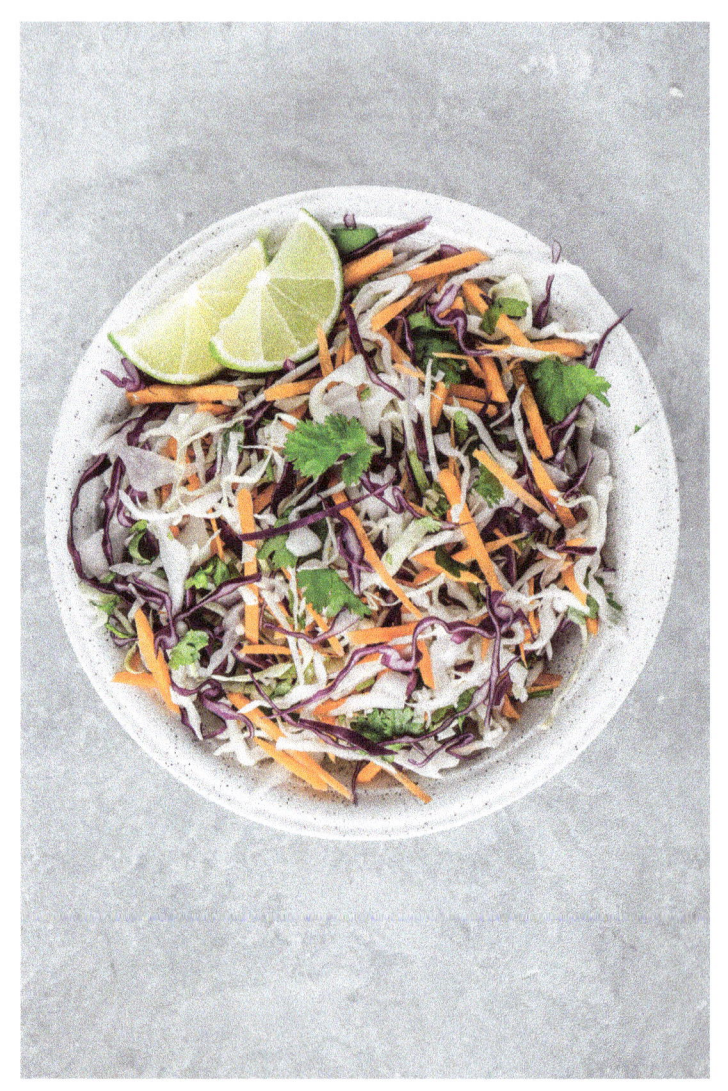

INSTRUCTIONS

1) Chop up all the veggies to roughly equal bite-sized pieces.

2) Mix dressing together with a fork until smooth. Pour over veggies and stir.

3) Sprinkle sesame, sunflower or pumpkin seeds on top.

Broccoli, Apples and Grapes with Apple Cider Vinaigrette

For the Salad

2 heads of broccoli chopped to bite-size

2 apples cored and chopped into small cubes

1 cup seedless grapes, cut in half

1/2 cup dried cranberries or raisins

1/2 red onion, diced

1/4 cup sliced almonds

For the Cider Vinaigrette

1/4 cup apple cider vinegar or balsamic vinegar

2 Tablespoons maple syrup or agave nectar

2 Tablespoons olive oil

1 teaspoon fresh or dried green herbs like parsley, oregano, basil

1/2 teaspoon garlic powder

1/2 teaspoon onion powder, *optional*

pinch of salt to taste

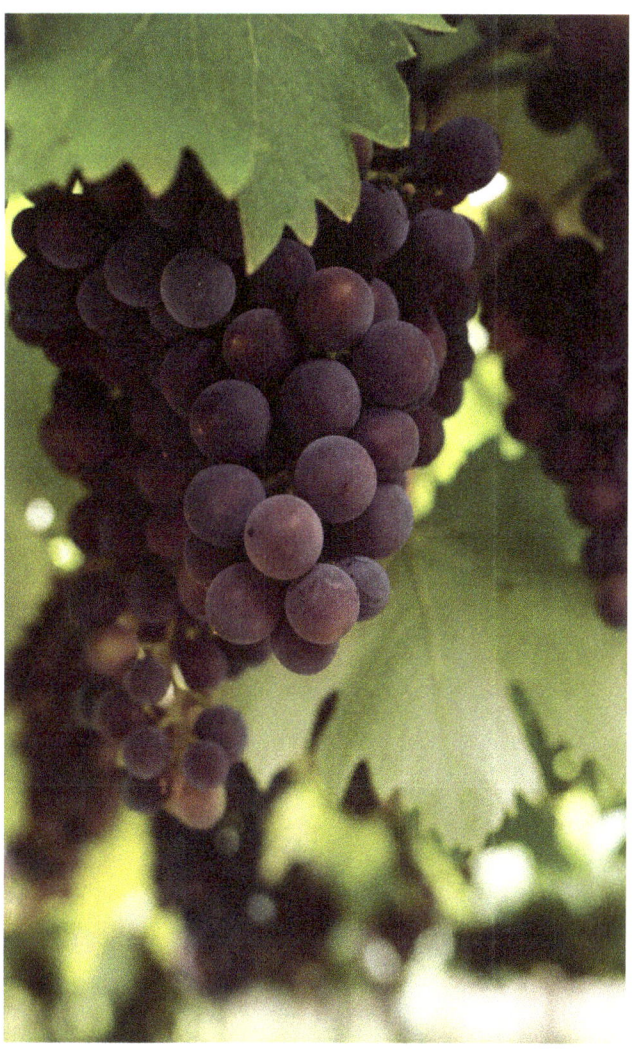

INSTRUCTIONS

1) Chop up the broccoli into small, bite-sized pieces. Chop the apple into small cubes. Chop onion into fine spears. Cut the grapes in half.

2) Mix all veggies with the almonds and cranberries/raisins.

3) Mix all cider vinaigrette ingredients with a fork and pour over salad. Stir.

Shaved Brussels Sprouts with Cranberries and Almonds

Servings: 5

For the Salad
1 lb. Brussels sprouts, trimmed and sliced thinly
1/2 cup dried, sweetened cranberries
1/4 cup sliced almonds or sunflower seeds
(*optional: toast almonds for extra flavor*)

For the Dressing
1/4 cup olive oil
1/8 cup lemon juice
1 Tablespoon Dijon mustard
1.5 Tablespoons maple syrup
1 teaspoon salt
1/2 teaspoon black pepper
1 teaspoon dried or fresh parsley

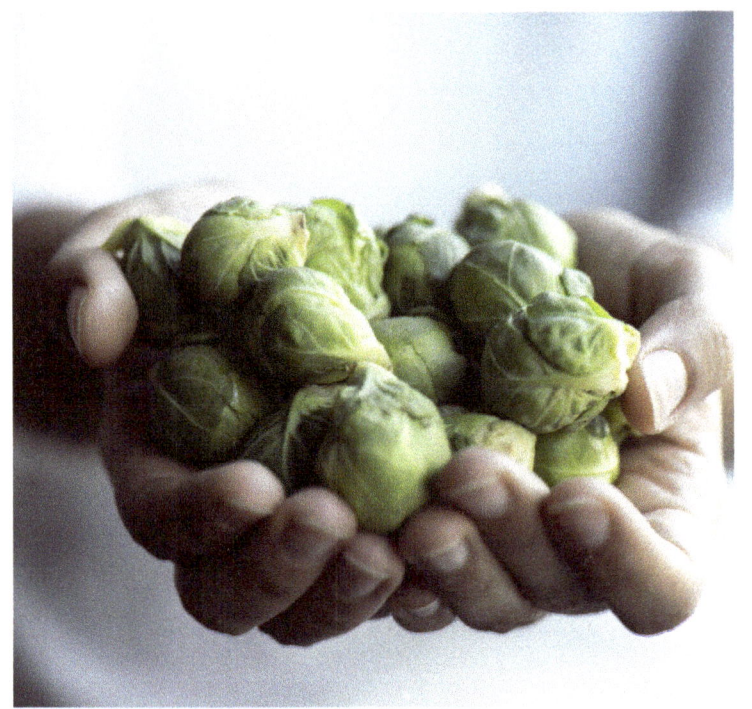

INSTRUCTIONS

1) Trim the hard stem end off of each Brussels sprout.

2) Cut each Brussels sprout in half and place the cut side down on a cutting board. Slice very thin (about 1/8 inch thick.) Put the sprouts in a medium bowl.

3) In a Mason jar, combine all other ingredients except for the almonds/sunflower seeds and cranberries. Stir and shake well to combine. Pour the dressing over the Brussels sprouts and mix well.

4) Add dried cranberries and sliced almonds and mix again.

Mason Jar Salad

A Mason Jar Salad can be made with any ingredients you have! Use a quart jar for a salad that will fill a bowl. The key to a delicious salad that can be stored for three days is to layer the ingredients in the jar from hardest to softest, with the hardest placed on the bottom layer with the dressing. These measurements are approximate; adjust them to your preferred proportions and ingredients.

For the Dressing

1 Tablespoon balsamic vinegar

1 Tablespoon olive oil

1 teaspoon or Tablespoon maple syrup, honey or agave nectar

a splash of fresh lemon juice

For the Salad

a half cup of chopped red cabbage

a quarter cup of chopped carrots

a half cup of chopped bell peppers or zucchini noodles

a few cherry tomatoes

a half cup of seasoned cooked beans, tofu, or tempeh

1/8 to 1/4 cup of nuts or seeds

a big handful of mixed leafy baby greens

INSTRUCTIONS

1) Pour the dressing into the jar first, then add hard, crunchy veggies like carrots and cabbage.

2) Above that layer, add softer veggies like chopped bell peppers, cherry tomatoes, and zucchini noodles.

3) Above that layer, add any protein you like, such as beans, tofu, tempeh, nuts, and seeds (and add avocado if you'll eat the salad the same day).

4) Finally, add your mixed leafy greens. When you're ready to eat, pour the salad out in a wide bowl, mix and enjoy.

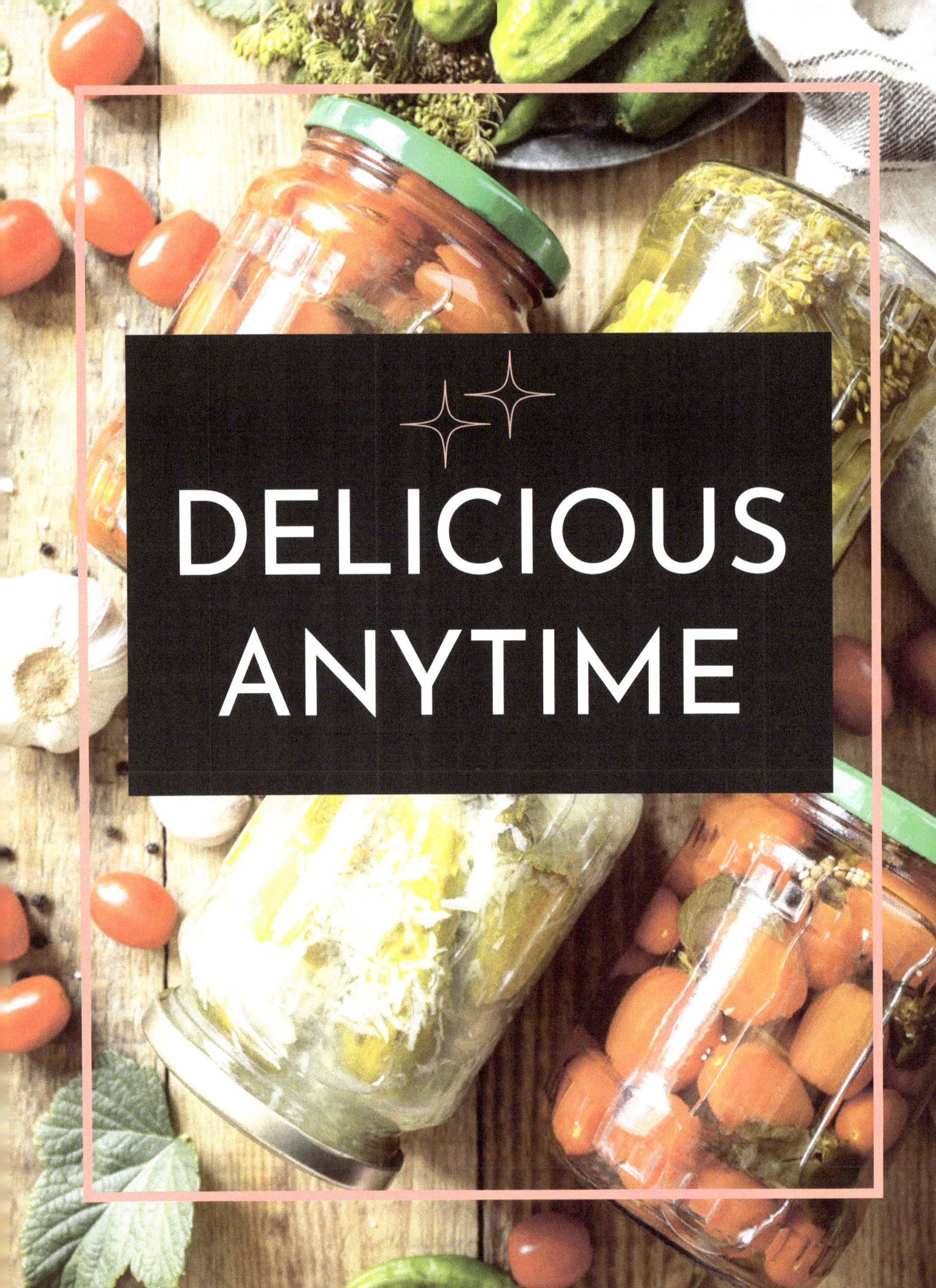

Crispy Baked Tofu

Servings: 5

Tofu is an incredible shape-shifter and can take on any flavor. I often cut a block in half longways into two flat slabs, marinate and eat them raw. Fears of soy intake increasing breast cancer risk have been thoroughly disproven; in fact, soy now appears to be a protective food.

The single most important key for making great tofu is to use a tofu press, which you can get for about $20. It presses several tablespoons of water out of a block of tofu in a few minutes, allowing it to absorb sauces and seasonings perfectly. You can also press tofu with something heavy like a brick or a cast iron skillet, if you wrap the tofu in a dishtowel and put it on a slanted cutting board... but a simple tofu press releases more water with less work.

- 2 blocks tofu
- 4 Tablespoons olive oil
- 4 Tablespoons tamari or soy sauce
- 4 Tablespoons arrowroot powder or cornstarch
- 1 teaspoon dried basil
- 1/2 teaspoon each of ginger powder, onion powder, garlic powder, oregano, and chile powder

INSTRUCTIONS

1) Squeeze/drain/press the blocks of tofu so they drain their extra water. Chop in bite-sized cubes. Preheat the oven to 400° F.

2) Mix olive oil, tamari/soy sauce and arrowroot powder/cornstarch in a medium bowl with any other herbs or spices you like.

3) Toss the tofu cubes in the mixture till they are well coated.

4) Line a baking tray with parchment paper or a silicon liner. Spread the tofu in one layer on a baking tray. Pour the rest of the sauce over the tofu, or save it for when you eat.

5) Bake for 25-30 minutes. Toss and turn the tofu halfway through so all sides get crispy.

Falafel Patties

Servings: 4-6

These tasty falafel patties are baked rather than fried for a healthier meal. When you are frying falafel, use chickpeas that are soaked, but not cooked. When you are baking falafel, use cooked chickpeas. These will keep nicely for a week refrigerated in a glass container.

- 3 cups chickpeas, cooked, or two cans chickpeas, drained and rinsed
- 1 medium yellow or red onion
- 4 cloves garlic
- 4 teaspoons coriander
- 1 teaspoon dried parsley
- 1 Tablespoon cold water
- 1-2 teaspoons cumin, to taste
- 1 Tablespoon arrowroot powder or flour
- 1/2 teaspoon salt
- 1/2 cup finely chopped fresh parsley, *optional*

INSTRUCTIONS

1) If cooking, soak 1 cup of dried chickpeas (garbanzo beans) overnight. Drain, rinse, and transfer to a pot. Cover with water twice the amount of beans and bring to a boil. Cover the pot, lower the heat and simmer for approximately one hour. Taste to make sure they're tender–if not, cook longer. Drain when they are done. If pressure cooking, add one part beans to two parts water and cook for 12 minutes on high with a 10-minute natural release.

2) Preheat oven to 375°F. Combine all the ingredients in the bowl of a food processor and process till creamy.

3) Prepare a baking tray with parchment paper or a silicon liner. Scoop out handfuls of the mixture and shape into twelve balls. Press onto the tray so they become patties.

4) Bake for 10 minutes, then flip falafel patties with a spatula. Bake for another 10-12 minutes.

5) Let patties cool so they hold their shape. Store them in a glass container. When you are ready to eat them, warm 1 Tablespoon oil in a pan and lightly cook them on each side so they brown and get a little crispy. They may be a slightly crumbly.

Cashew Queso

This recipe is adapted from The Minimalist Baker. It is wonderful with corn chips, carrot sticks, or over nachos.

- 3/4 – 1 cup hot water
- 1 cup raw cashews, dry or soaked for 4 to 8 hours (if soaked, start with 1/2 cup water)
- 1 clove garlic, chopped
- 2 Tablespoons nutritional yeast
- 1/2 teaspoon ground cumin
- 1 teaspoon chili powder
- 1/2 teaspoon salt, plus more to taste
- 1 Tablespoon hot salsa, hot sauce or harissa

INSTRUCTIONS

1) Add all ingredients to a high-speed blender, Nutribullet blender or food processor, starting with 3/4 cup of water. Blend until creamy, adding more water as needed. Add just enough water to achieve a creamy, pourable queso. If it gets too thin, thicken with more raw cashews.

2) Taste and adjust flavor as needed, adding more nutritional yeast for cheesiness, salt to taste, cumin for smokiness, chili powder or hot sauce for heat, or garlic for zing.

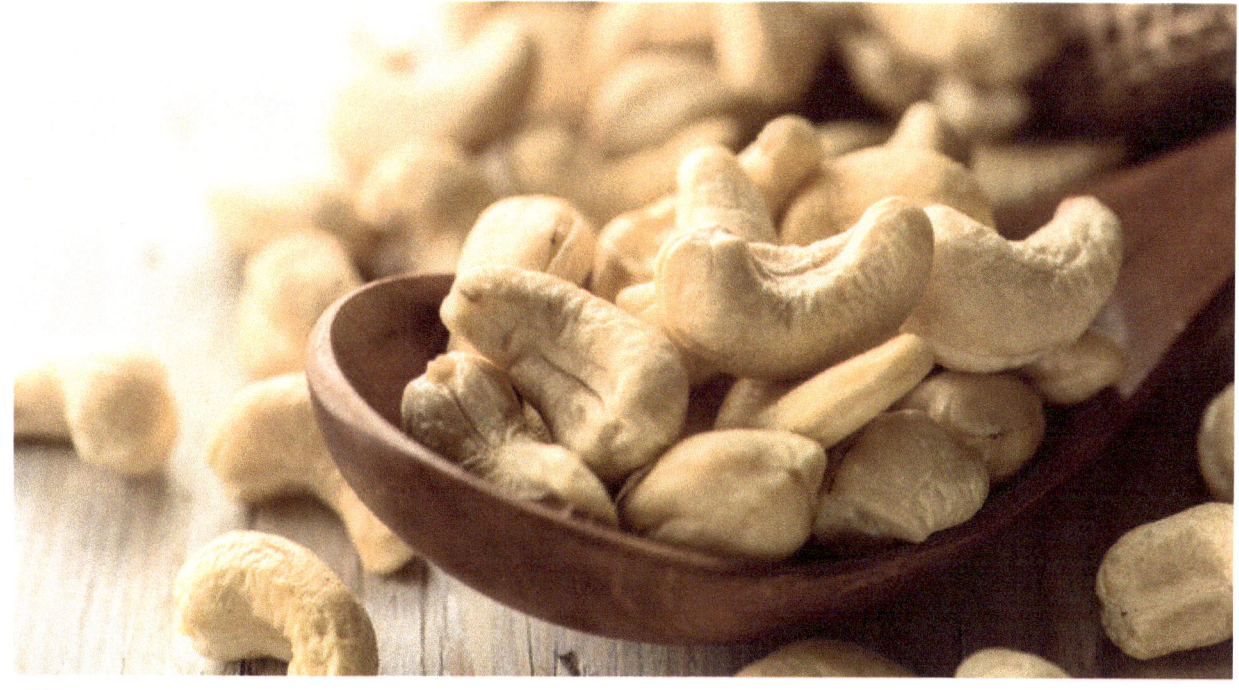

Bean Dip

Servings: 5

This is my go-to bean dip for parties and to serve as an appetizer on the table when I have hungry kids visiting. I serve it cold with carrot and celery sticks. It is a potent preventative medicine with raw garlic and lemon and is just the right amount of spicy to be refreshing.

- 1.5 cups cooked chickpeas (or 1 can, rinsed and drained)
- 1.5 cups cooked black beans (or 1 can, rinsed and drained)
- 1/4 cup sesame seeds
- 1 Tablespoon olive oil
- 1/4 cup lemon juice
- 1/4 cup water
- 1 garlic clove
- 1 teaspoon ground cumin
- 1/2 teaspoon crushed red pepper
- 1/2 teaspoon salt, to taste

INSTRUCTIONS

1) Place all ingredients into a high-speed blender and firmly secure the lid.

2) Start the blender and slowly increase to highest speed.

3) Blend for 50 seconds or until a smooth consistency is reached.

4) Pour the bean dip into glass container. Serve with raw carrots and celery.

Perfect Collards

Servings: 4

These collard greens have only six ingredients and come together in less than ten minutes for a taste-bud exalting side dish with the curative power of cruciferous vegetables.

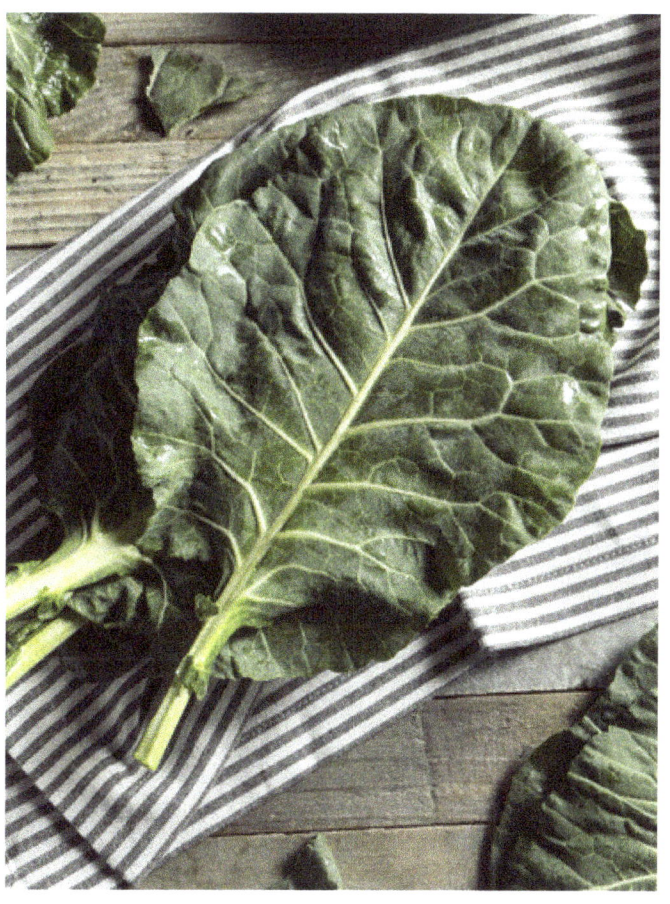

- 2-3 bunches collard greens
- 1 medium red onion
- 1 Tablespoon olive oil
- 1 Tablespoon balsamic vinegar
- 1 Tablespoon tamari or soy sauce
- 1 Tablespoon maple syrup

INSTRUCTIONS

1) Cut two or three bunches of collard greens into ribbons, slicing the greens off the spine first, then cutting each piece into smaller strips. Chop the red onion into thin spears.

2) In a large pan, add olive oil and sauté the onion for 5 minutes, then add the chopped collard greens, stir, and put a cover on the pan for 2 minutes.

3) Mix together vinegar, tamari, and maple syrup. Pour over the collard greens and stir. Cook to desired tenderness—just a few minutes more. If you'd like more saturated greens, add more tamari, vinegar and maple syrup.

Spicy Quick-Pickled Veggies

This dish is a variation on the Latin American dish *escabeche*, spicy picked vegetables served as a condiment. The recipe can be made entirely with carrots as the hard vegetable or can be varied with a ratio of 1/2 carrots, 1/4 yams and 1/4 cauliflower. This simple refrigerator pickle is easy to make and beautiful in a jar. It will last for up to a month in the fridge. I eat it as a healthy snack and add it to pastas and sandwiches for a kick of flavor.

2 pounds of hard vegetables, like carrots, yams, cauliflower
1/2 cup jalapeños, sliced
1/2 cup white or red onion, sliced
5 cloves garlic, smashed
2.5 cups white vinegar
2.5 cups water

1 Tablespoon vegetable oil
6 bay leaves
10 black peppercorns
2 teaspoons dried oregano
2 teaspoons sugar, *optional*
1 teaspoon salt

INSTRUCTIONS

1) Slice carrots on the diagonal into round coins (not into sticks), about 1/2 to 1/2 inch thick. Slice yams into rounds the same thickness, and then chop the rounds into six parts to get pieces of yam about the same size as the carrots. Slice cauliflower into small bite-sized pieces.

2) In a large stock pot, combine vinegar, water, bay leaves, peppercorns, oregano, salt and sugar (if using).

3) Bring the solution to a boil and add carrots, jalapeños, onions and any other vegetables you are including.

4) Lower heat to medium-low and cook for 15 minutes, uncovered.

5) Turn off heat and allow the liquid and vegetables to cool for at least half an hour.

6) When the pot is cool to the touch, use a steel jar funnel and a ladle to pour vegetables and liquid into glass Mason jars. Make sure to get a good mix of veggies in each jar. If more liquid is needed than you have in the stock pot, add equal parts vinegar and water. (You can also store this in Tupperware or square glass containers.)

7) Close up the Mason jars with lids. You can eat it at any time! The flavors will really marry well after three hours. Store it in the refrigerator for up to a month. In a jar, it also makes a lovely gift for neighbors.

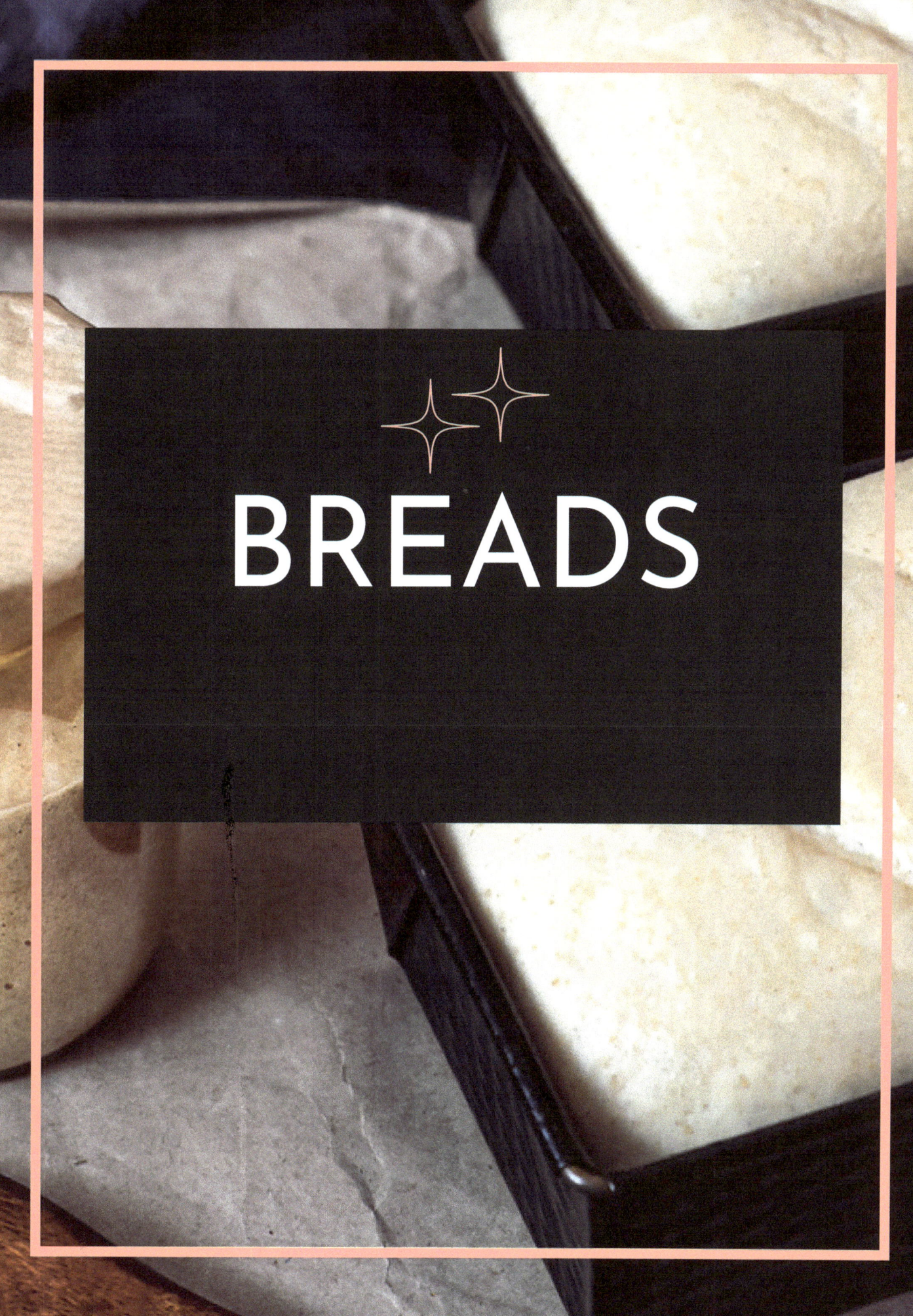

BREADS

Cornbread in a Cast Iron Skillet

Servings: 12

This cornbread showcases the amazing depth and versatility of maize. It's a Northern cornbread because it is unsweetened–but has pecans for a Southern touch.

- 1 cup yellow cornmeal
- 1/2 teaspoon salt
- 1/2 teaspoon baking soda
- 1 cup nondairy milk
- 1 flax egg (1 Tablespoon flaxseed powder + 3 Tablespoons water, mixed)
- 1 cup fresh or frozen, thawed corn kernels
- 1/4 cup pecans
- 2 teaspoons olive oil

INSTRUCTIONS

1) Preheat the oven to 450°F.

2) In medium bowl, mix the cornmeal, salt, and baking soda. In a small bowl, mix together the flax egg–let it sit for a few minutes to thicken. Add the nondairy milk. Combine milk and flax mixture with cornmeal mixture. Stir in the corn kernels. Mix with a few strokes, but not excessively.

3) Heat a 10-inch cast iron skillet for 5 minutes in the oven. When skillet is hot, add the oil and swirl it around. Pour the batter in the pan. Add the pecans on top in a pretty pattern. Bake for 10 minutes or until knife inserted in the center comes out clean. Cool for 5 minutes in the pan. Serve warm drizzled with maple syrup or alongside a hearty soup.

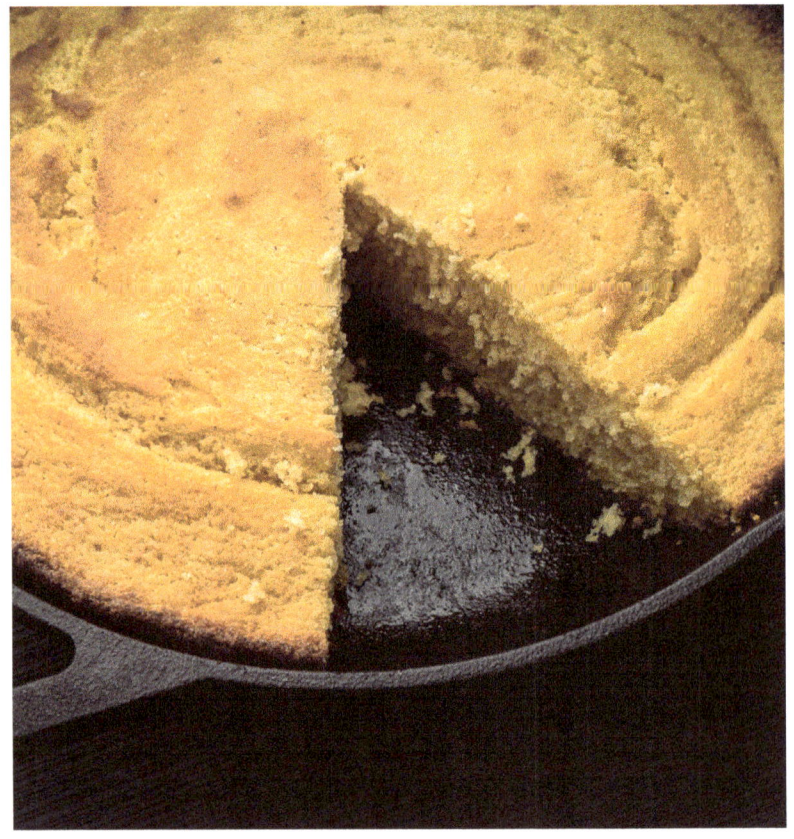

Children's Bread

Servings: 16

This bread is legendary in my childhood. My mother named it "children's bread" because it's so easy that children can make it, starting at about age six (with help using the oven). We would sit on the floor with a big silver mixing bowl to pour the ingredients and stir, then *ooh* and *ahh* as the dough rose like magic. Children feel extremely accomplished when they make this bread! Adults do, too. I normally wouldn't use white flour but make an exception here of half white and half whole wheat flour because it is so delicious.

- 3 cups hot water
- 2/3 cup honey (or molasses for a vegan version)
- 3 cups white flour
- 1 package yeast
- 3 cups whole wheat flour

INSTRUCTIONS

1) Mix hot water, honey, and white flour in a large bowl. Add yeast and whole wheat flour and mix again.

2) Let rise in a warm place for 1 hour, covered by a damp dishtowel.

3) Stir the dough down. Pour it into 2 greased loaf pans. Let it rise 15 minutes more. Preheat the oven to 350°F.

3) Put the loaf pans in the oven and bake for one hour. If the bread is getting too brown on top, cover with a sheet of tin foil.

4) Remove from oven and let cool. Slice and serve with vegan butter and raw honey. It cuts more cleanly the next day.

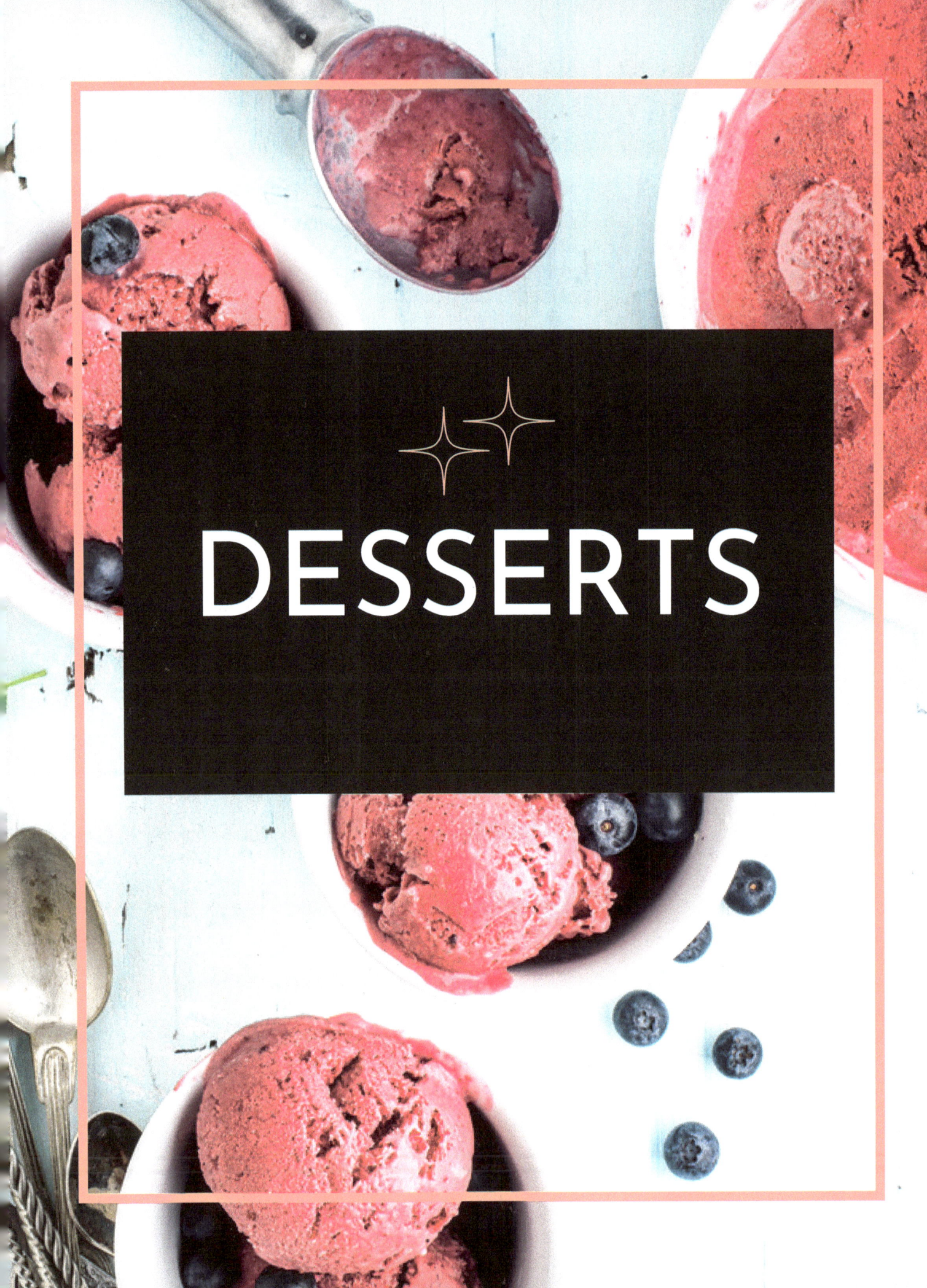

DESSERTS

Veronica's Haroset

Servings: 6

This is my mother's recipe for a traditional Jewish dish served at Passover. It is so scrumptious and refreshing it can be enjoyed anytime as a dessert fruit salad. It gives a powerful boost of antioxidants in the warming spices.

- 6 apples, grated
- 3 Tablespoons honey (or agave nectar for a vegan version)
- 1/4 cup sweet red wine, such as Manischewitz fruit wine
- 1 teaspoon cinnamon
- 1/2 cup chopped pecans
- 1/8 teaspoon cloves
- 1/8 teaspoon nutmeg

INSTRUCTIONS

1) In a large bowl, grate the apples with their skins on or off, as you prefer.

2) Chop the pecans to small pieces.

2) Mix apples, pecans, wine, and spices and stir. Serve in bowls or on a flat wheat cracker with a little bit of horseradish spread.

Coconut Jicama Salad

Servings: 4

This dessert fruit salad works with lots of variations. If you don't have jicama, you can use any other hard fruit like pear or apple.

- 1 medium jicama, peeled and cut in small strips (julienned)
- 1/2 cup seedless grapes, cut in half, *optional*
- 2 kiwis, peeled and cut in thin rounds or cubes
- 1/3 cup shredded or shaved coconut
- 1/2 orange with segments chopped in thirds
- Juice of the other half of the orange poured over salad
- 1 teaspoon sesame seeds

INSTRUCTIONS

1) Chop jicama, grapes, kiwis and half an orange.

2) Mix in a medium bowl. Add the coconut and sesame seeds. Squeeze the juice of the other half of the orange over the fruit and mix well with a spoon. Chill.

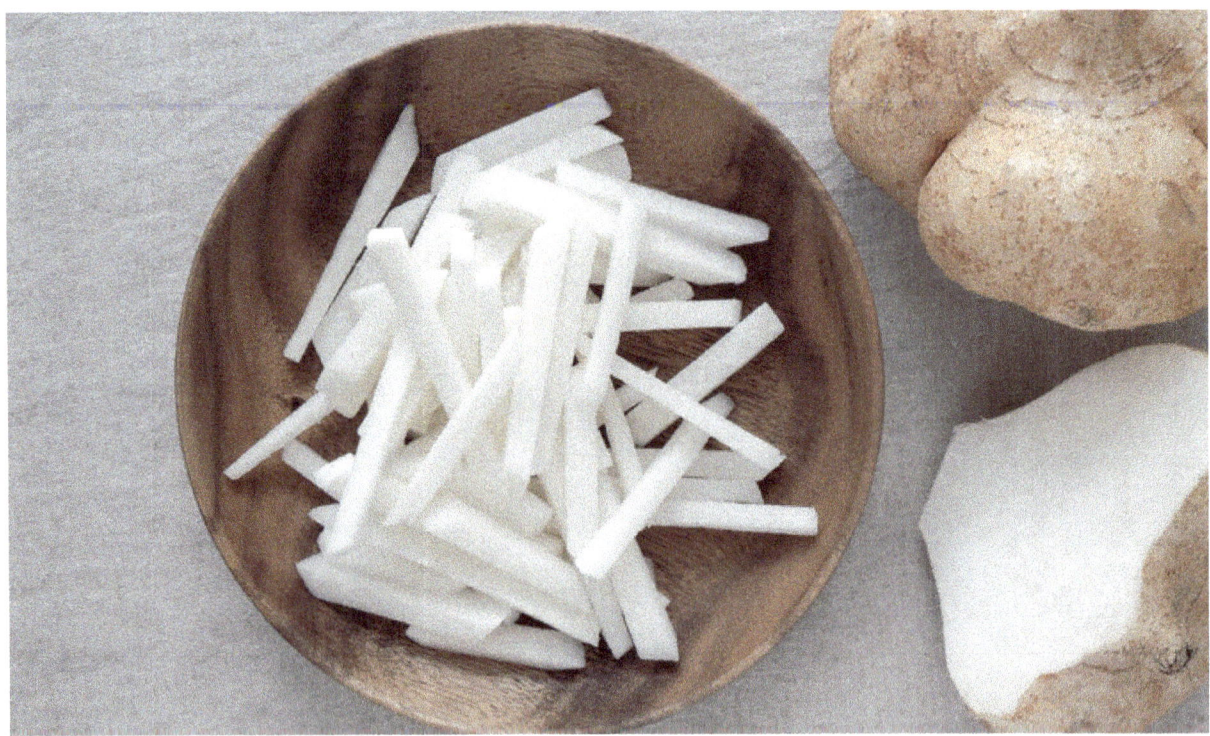

Mango, Pomegranate, Blueberry Salad

Servings: 5

This fruit salad invented by my friend is incredibly simple and visually stunning—the yellow, red and blue palette makes a striking display. I like to bring it to parties, where it gets quickly devoured.

- 4 to 6 fresh mangos, peeled and sliced
- 1 cup pomegranate seeds
- 1 cup fresh blueberries
- juice of one lime

INSTRUCTIONS

1) Peel and slice mangoes.

2) Arrange this salad on a platter so that the mangos are in a single layer, rather than in a bowl. Sprinkle the blueberries and pomegranate seeds on top and squeeze the juice of one lime over the platter. Voila!

Oatmeal Pecan Date Balls

Servings: 12 (1 per serving)

I like to keep these around at all times for snacking on as well as feeding guests and kids. They're deceptively satisfying and not too-too sweet.

- 1.5 cups soft pitted dates
- 1 cup rolled oats
- 1 cup pecans
- 2 Tablespoons brown sugar
- 1 flax egg (1 Tablespoon ground flaxseeds mixed with 2 Tablespoons water, allowed to sit for a few minutes)
- 1.5 teaspoons ground cinnamon
- 1 teaspoon vanilla extract
- pinch of salt

INSTRUCTIONS

1) Combine the dates, pecans, and oats in a food processor and process until the mixture is crumbly.

2) Add the brown sugar, flax egg, cinnamon and vanilla and process again, until the dough sticks together. If it's too dry, add 1 teaspoon water at a time.

3) Line a baking sheet with parchment paper or a silicon mat. Scoop out about a Tablespoon of the dough and roll it between your palms until it makes a ball. Make all the dough into balls and fill the sheet. If you like, you can press a fork into the balls to flatten them a bit. Refrigerate for three to four hours before serving.

Spiced Berry Sorbet

Servings: 4

Berries and spices are so full of antioxidants that to me, they qualify as medicinal food. This delicious easy dessert leaves me full of energy after a meal. In the heat of summer, it's good to rejuvenate with sorbet.

- 1 finger of fresh ginger root, peeled
- 1 cup cold water
- 3/4 cup granulated sugar
- 6 cups frozen berries thawed for 15 minutes
- 1/2 teaspoon ground cinnamon
- 1/4 teaspoon ground nutmeg
- 1/8 teaspoon ground cloves
- 1/8 teaspoon ground allspice
- 1 teaspoon vanilla extract

INSTRUCTIONS

1) Add ginger, sugar and water into a high-speed blender and secure the lid. Start blender and slowly increase to medium speed. Blend for 25 seconds until ginger is finely chopped.

2) Add berries, cinnamon, nutmeg, cloves, allspice, and vanilla. Secure the lid. Start blender and slowly increase to highest speed. Blend for 1 minute, using tamper to press ingredients into blades if necessary.

3) Pour sorbet into cups and enjoy. Put any unused sorbet into a glass container, label and freeze for later.

Cucumber Jalapeño Popsicles

Servings: 4-6

Adjust the spices and sweetness level on this refreshing summer popsicle to your pleasure.

- 1.5 cups cucumber, peeled and chopped
- 1.5 cups coconut water
- 1/4 cup lemon juice
- 1/2 of a green jalapeño pepper, seeds removed (*optional: add in 5-20 seeds for a spicier popsicle*)
- 2 Tablespoons honey or 10 drops liquid stevia or 2 Tablespoons maple syrup
- 1/2 teaspoon wheatgrass or spirulina powder, *optional*

INSTRUCTIONS

1) Blend all ingredients in a high-speed blender.

2) Strain the solids out using a mesh strainer.

3) Pour the liquid into popsicle molds and freeze.

Thumbprint Cookies

Servings: 24-30 cookies

This is a whole foods plant based variation on the classic thumbprint cookie. They're just sweet enough to satisfy the taste buds and feel decadent. Experiment with the fillings, or leave out the spices for a more traditional-tasting cookie. This recipe is adapted from the cookbook *One Bite at a Time*.

- 1 cup raw almonds
- 1 cup rolled oats
- 1 cup all-purpose flour or spelt flour
- 1/2 teaspoon ground cinnamon
- 1/4 teaspoon ground ginger
- 1/8 teaspoon ground cardamom
- 1/8 teaspoon ground nutmeg
- 1/4 teaspoon salt
- 1/2 cup olive, safflower or canola oil
- 1/2 cup maple syrup (increase to taste)
- 1/2 teaspoon vanilla extract
- Jam, for filling cookies

INSTRUCTIONS

1) Preheat the oven to 350° F and line a baking sheet with parchment paper or a silicon liner.

2) In a food processor or blender, grind the almonds into a coarse flour for about 2 minutes. Add the oats, flour, spices, and salt and process for another minute.

3) Add the oil, maple syrup and vanilla extract. Process for 1 to 2 minutes more until combined. The dough will form into a ball. Wrap the dough in plastic wrap or a beeswax wrap and let it sit at room temperature for 10 minutes to cohere.

4) Roll 1 Tablespoon of the dough into a ball between your palms, place it on the prepared cookie sheet and press your thumb or the back of a spoon into the center of each cookie. Fill it with your favorite jam or marmalade (or experiment with chocolate chips, peanut butter or other fillings.)

5) Place all the cookies on the sheet about an inch apart. Bake for 15 minutes, or until their bottoms are lightly browned. Enjoy!

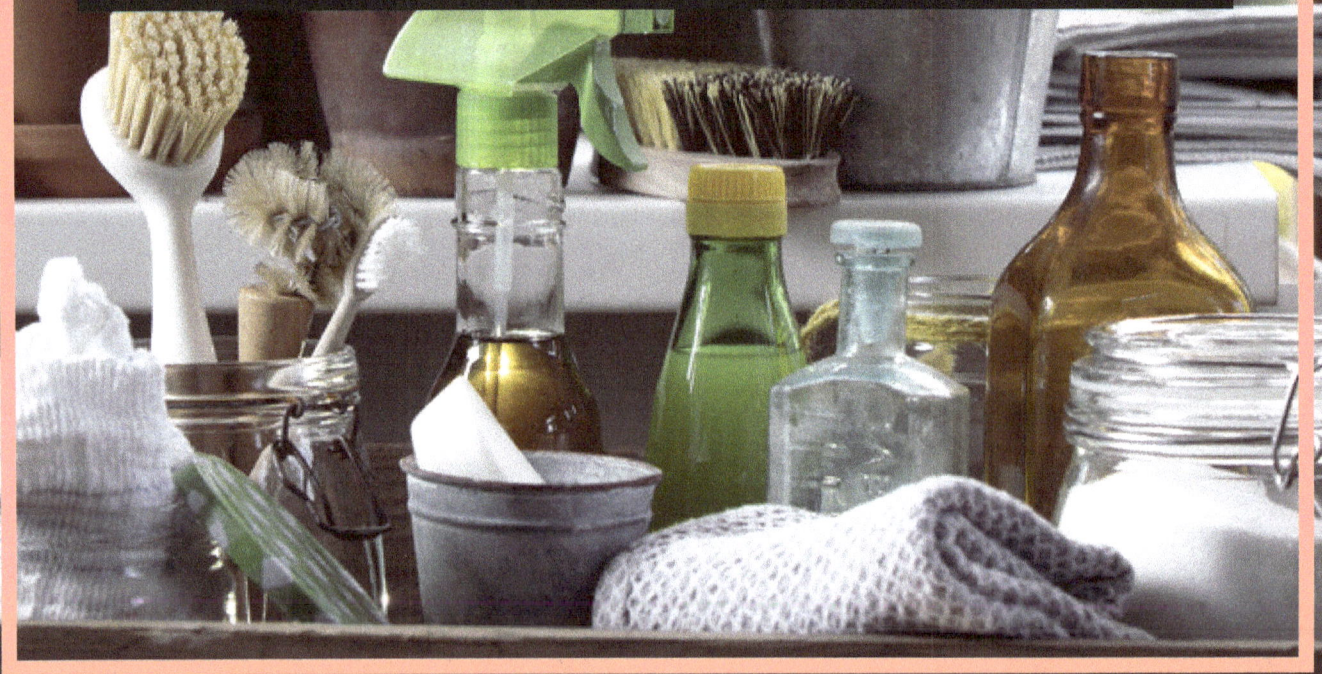

BODY CARE & CLEANING

Body Care Recipes

Here are some other delights that I keep at home in glass jars. The measurements can be inexact– play around and see what smells you like!

A good starter essential oil pantry kit will contain peppermint, lemongrass, orange, lavender, rose, cedar, eucalyptus, and rosemary.

MOUTHWASH

Combine in a glass jar or bottle:

- 3 cups filtered water
- 2 Tablespoons baking soda
- 20 drops peppermint essential oil
- salt to taste
- 1 teaspoon calcium citrate powder to strengthen teeth, *optional*

DEODORANT

Combine in a glass spray bottle or an old spray deodorant bottle:

- 1 cup isopropyl alcohol, grain alcohol or high-proof vodka
- 1/4 cup filtered water
- 20 drops of one essential oil (lavender, rose, rosemary are good options)

or

- 1 cup pure witch hazel
- 1/4 cup grain alcohol, isopropyl alcohol or high-proof vodka
- 20 drops of one essential oil of your choice

MOISTURIZING ROSEWATER SPRITZ

Combine in an atomizing spray bottle:

- 2 cups filtered water
- 2 teaspoons glycerin
- 20 drops rose essential oil

Spritz your face and torso to activate your heart chakra.

SUGAR SCRUB

- 1/3 cup olive oil
- 4 Tablespoons honey
- 1 cup sugar (white or raw/turbinado)
- 10 drops essential oil of your choice

Combine in pint-sized Mason jar, stir well, close up and put a bow on it. Makes a lovely exfoliating body and face scrub that also moisturizes deeply, and is a nice gift.

BATH SALTS

- 2 cups Epsom salts
- 30 drops essential oil (eucalyptus, cedar, lavender, or rosemary)

Combine in a bowl, stir well, then pour into a pint jar and decorate with a ribbon. If using a half-pint jar, halve the recipe.

HAND AND FACE LOTION

- 1/2 cup almond oil (or sunflower, or olive)
- 1/4 cup coconut oil
- 1/8 cup beeswax
- 1 tablespoon shea butter (or cocoa butter)
- 20 drops lavender essential oil (or rose, tea tree, or your favorite scent)
- 1 teaspoon Vitamin E oil (to preserve the lotion)

Combine the first four ingredients in a pint (medium) wide mouth Mason jar. You will add essential oil and Vitamin E later.

Place jar into a saucepan and add enough water to the pan so that the water level is higher than the ingredients in the jar (don't add water to the jar, just the pan.) Heat the water on medium low and allow the ingredients to slowly melt inside the jar. This can take 10 to 20 minutes.

Once the ingredients are melted, remove the pan from heat and place the jar on a towel or heat-safe surface. Let it cool for a few minutes.

Add essential oils and Vitamin E. Gently stir to combine. Pour the salve into a half-pint wide mouth Mason jar with a lid. If you want it to set up more quickly, place in fridge for an hour. Store at room temperature.

Cleaning Supply Recipes

EVERYDAY CLEANING SPRAY

Combine in a jar with a trigger spray top:

- 2 cups water
- 2 cups white vinegar
- 20 drops citrus essential oil

BRIGHTENING LAUNDRY SOAP

- 2 cups Borax
- 2 cups washing soda (not baking soda)
- 2 cups finely grated Castile soap flakes
- 30 drops of one essential oil of your choice (lemon, orange, lavender)

Combine ingredients and mix in a bowl, then pour into a half-gallon jar. Use 1/4 cup per load, adding to the washing machine water before adding clothes.

GLASS CLEANER

Combine in a jar with a trigger spray top:

- 1 cup water
- 1 cup rubbing alcohol (70% concentration)
- 1/2 cup white vinegar
- 1 to 2 drops of a citrus essential oil for scent (optional)

Spray solution on a microfiber cloth or plain black-and-white newspaper to clean windows and mirrors.

Acknowledgments

Thank you for going on this tour of magical food and the Mason jar life, a peaceful kitchen system. I hope that you are inspired to try batch cooking and build a jar library of your own. Have lots of potluck dinner parties. Practice simplicity and tender loving care for yourself. May your health and happiness flourish!

I am grateful to all the people who have taught me to cook over my lifetime, who have shared meals at their tables, and who have taught me compassion and care for living beings. I am especially grateful to my mother, whose kitchen is a marvel of jars and whose heart is a kaliedoscope of love. After her kitchen, I learned to cook first at the New Orleans Zen Center as a resident student, then at Tenney House Vegetarian Collective dorm at Smith College, and then at the festive feminist holiday celebrations at Deep Dish in Albion, in the Northern California redwood forest. I'm still learning how to cook from each vegetarian cookbook I come across. I cherish every opportunity to prepare food and celebrate life with loved ones and new friends, and humbly thank everyone who has broken bread and told stories with me.

Thanks to all those friends who encouraged me to share this peaceful kitchen system just a few months ago. Thanks to my close readers of early drafts, liz moseley, Maxfield Bell and Erin Burrows; to Caitlyn Perdue and Laurel Barickman for beautiful designs; to Cynthia Frank for mentoring and to Kristin Harrison for mindset coaching.

I write this with gratitude from Austin, Texas which is unceded territory of the Tonkawa people, also occupied and passed through by the Alabama-Coushatta, Caddo, Carrizo/Comecrudo, Coahuiltecan, Comanche, Kickapoo, Lipan Apache, and Ysleta Del Sur Pueblo peoples.

My prayer is that by changing how we eat, and choosing with loving intention how we relate to the Earth and all her living beings, including people, animals, fish, birds, insects, trees, food plants, medicine plants, weeds, water, air, and soil, we can continue to live here together long enough to heal what has fallen out of balance, and partake fully in the miracle of life, as the peaceful caretakers we are meant to be.

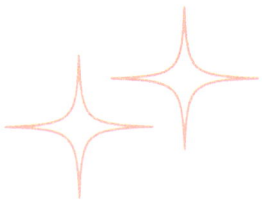

Recommended Reading

The Blue Zones Kitchen: 100 Recipes to Live to 100
by Dan Buettner
Immersing himself in the 5 regions of the world where people live the longest, the author distilled health principles and collected their recipes. These plant-based dishes are mouthwatering, the recipes are perfect and the commentary is fascinating.

Eat Plants, Bitch! 91 Vegan Recipes that Will Blow Your Meat-Loving Mind
by Pinky Cole
Chef Pinky Cole is known as The Slutty Vegan, doyenne of vegan comfort food. She gathers advice from Black vegan chefs and offers her own healthy, soul-food inflected dishes you won't find in other cookbooks.

How Not to Die
by Dr. Michael Greger
A dazzling tour-de-force of research about the foods that cause, prevent and heal the most common disease- and lifestyle-based causes of death in the modern world.

The How Not to Die Cookbook
by Dr. Michael Greger
I turn to this cookbook more than any other for perfectly-tuned recipes that maximize nutrient-dense whole foods.

In the Green Kitchen: Techniques to Learn by Heart
by Alice Waters
From simmering beans to wilting greens, steaming vegetables to baking fruit, the veteran natural chef gives virtuosic lessons and recipes.

The Korean Vegan: Reflections and Recipes from Omma's Kitchen
by Joanne Lee Molinaro
Instagram sensation @thekoreanvegan is a spellbinding storyteller and incredible cook. For example, her Chocolate Sweet Potato Cake recipe is an homage to the two foods that saved her mother's life after she fled North Korea.

Power Plates: 100 Nutritionally Balanced, One-Dish Vegan Meals
by Gena Hamshaw
It can be strenuous to figure out if you're getting the right mix of macronutrients (protein, fat and carbohydrates) every day, and this cookbook presents one-bowl meals that have those proportions perfectly balanced for health and flavor.

About the Author

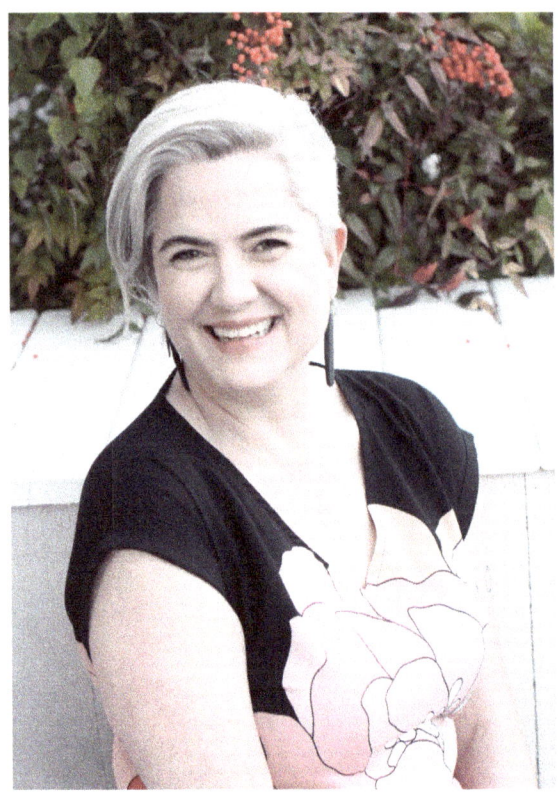

Abe Louise Young is a writer and educator who believes in a world where beings of every species can live peacefully. Her work has been published in The Nation, The New York Times, Poetry Magazine, New Letters, Narrative Magazine and elsewhere. She's the author of three collections of poetry and various guides for educators and youth advocates. She love playing around in the kitchen, weaving community connections, talking to strangers and feeding her friends and family. Connect with her at abelouiseyoung.com.

www.ingramcontent.com/pod-product-compliance
Lightning Source LLC
Chambersburg PA
CBHW061821290426
44110CB00027B/2934